SONOGRAPHY IN GYNECOLOGY AND OBSTETRICS

Just the Facts

SONOGRAPHY IN GYNECOLOGY AND OBSTETRICS

Just the Facts

Arthur C. Fleischer, M.D.

Professor of Radiology and Radiological Sciences
Professor of Obstetrics and Gynecology
Chief of Diagnostic Sonography
Vanderbilt University Medical Center
Nashville, Tennessee

McGRAW-HILL
Medical Publishing Division

New York   Chicago   San Francisco   Lisbon   London   Madrid
Mexico City   Milan   New Delhi   San Juan   Seoul   Singapore
Sydney   Toronto

Sonography in Gynecology and Obstetrics: *Just the Facts*

1 2 3 4 5 6 7 8 9 0   IMA/IMA   0 9 8 7 6 5 4 3

ISBN 0-07-141851-2

This book was set in Times New Roman by The GTS Companies/York, PA Campus.
The editor was Andrea Seils.
Project management was provided by Andover Publishing Services.
The production supervisor was Philip Galea.
The index was prepared by Andover Publishing Services.
The printer and binder was Imago (U.S.A.), Inc., Singapore.

This book is printed on acid-free paper.

Library of Congress Cataloging-in-Publication Data

Sonography in gynecology and obstetrics : just the facts / edited by Arthur C. Fleischer.
     p. ; cm.
  Includes bibliographical references and index.
  ISBN 0-07-141851-2
  1. Ultrasonics in obstetrics. 2. Generative organs, Female—Ultrasonic imaging. I. Fleischer, Arthur C.
  [DNLM: 1. Genital Diseases, Female—ultrasonography. 2. Pregnancy Complications—ultrasonography. 3. Ultrasonography—methods. WP 141 S699 2004]
  RG527.5.U48 S657
  618′.047543–dc21
                                                                                    2003044932

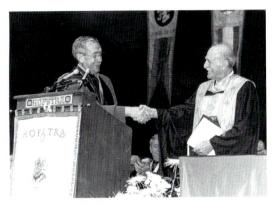

Professor Julian Kaufman (right) at his retirement ceremony.

Dedication

This book is dedicated to my parents, Gene and Lucille Fleischer, J.D.;
my late grand uncle, Julian Kaufman, M.F.A.;
and my grand aunt Lillian, in recognition of their lifelong encouragement
of my academic and clinical pursuits.

PREFACE

This book provides radiology and obstetrics/gynecology trainees with an informative overview of the fundamental principles used in diagnostic sonography (ultrasound) in gynecology and obstetrics. It will also be useful to sonography students and practicing sonographers, medical students, and other medical professionals who are dedicated to excellence in the practice of diagnostic sonography.

Sonography in Gynecology and Obstetrics: Just the Facts is derived from the larger, more encyclopedic textbook, *Sonography in Obstetrics and Gynecology: Principles and Practice,* 6th edition. This book is presented in abbreviated, outline form, and emphasizes the major principles used in clinical practice. More than 750 images and drawings, many in color, are provided to illustrate these fundamentals. While most of the images are taken from the larger textbook, about 90 images are new to this publication.

Each chapter contains a list of references, which refer to specific chapters in the textbook and to selected recently published scientific papers that are considered "landmark" works. The reader is encouraged to refer to the larger book for a more detailed discussion of particular topics of interest and for additional related references.

Because the use of diagnostic sonography in gynecology and obstetrics continues to expand as the technology improves, it challenges those of us who utilize sonography every day to come up with new clinical applications of this versatile diagnostic modality. This book is written with the hope that it will enable more patients to derive maximal clinical benefit from the dedicated health care professionals who utilize this wonderfully useful diagnostic modality to its fullest.

Arthur C. Fleischer, M.D.

ACKNOWLEDGMENTS

I express my gratitude to Andrea Seils, medical editor at McGraw-Hill, who has encouraged and skillfully guided the publication of this work, and to Vera Merriweather, my assistant, who has expertly prepared the numerous drafts of the text. I thank our sonography students and their director, Jill Herzog, RDMS, for their constructive criticisms of the book. I also express my appreciation to Marilyn D. Davis, RDMS, and her dedicated staff of sonographers, whose everyday efforts provide the best and most caring clinical service to our patients.

I also want to acknowledge all my clinical and research colleagues, who have provided great insight and creative zeal. And lastly, I want to thank Dominic Doyle and Paul Gross for their superb illustrations, which convey important concepts of sonographic imaging in gynecology and obstetrics.

SONOGRAPHY IN GYNECOLOGY AND OBSTETRICS

Just the Facts

1 INSTRUMENTATION AND SCANNING TECHNIQUES

OVERVIEW

- The proper and optimal use of diagnostic sonography requires a full working knowledge of the principles used to acquire and interpret sonographic images.
- This chapter describes the fundamental principles of the instrumentation and scanning techniques that will optimize the clinically useful information derived from sonography.
- Widely accepted guidelines for performing and interpreting gynecologic and obstetric sonography are included in the two appendixes at the end of the book.

IMPORTANT DEFINITIONS AND TERMS

- *Sonography*: the use of ultrasound (high-frequency pressure waves) for depicting anatomy and physiology; the images obtained reflect differences in acoustic impedance within tissues
- *Transducer*: electrical device used for sonographic imaging that detects differences in pressure or electrical charge
- *Probe*: scanning instrument that contains transducers used for sonographic imaging
- *Bioeffects*: biological effects of sonography, usually potential, on a patient, fetus, and/or sonographer

TYPES OF TRANSDUCERS/PROBES USED IN GYNECOLOGIC/OBSTETRIC SONOGRAPHY

TRANSVAGINAL PROBES

- Probes can be characterized by their "footprint" or scanning surface; the rounded shape of the probe housing optimizes manipulation of probe for transvaginal scanning (Fig. 1-1):
  - *Curvilinear*: contains hundreds of subelements arranged in a gently curving array; the subelements are activated and received according to electronic phasing
  - *Tight convex*: highest line density, smallest footprint—subelements are arranged in a semicircular array
  - *Mechanical sector*: single or multiple (up to three) rotating or oscillating transducers that display a sector field-of-view
  - *Linear array*: transducer subelements are arranged in a linear configuration that is displayed in a rectangular field-of-view

TRANSABDOMINAL PROBES

- *Curvilinear* probes give the largest field-of-view, and provide an elongated sector field-of-view.
- *Linear array* probes are good for imaging large areas or superficial structures or providing uniform compression over structures such as the area of the appendix (Fig. 1-2).
- *Sector array* probes have a relatively small footprint, and are good for intercostal scanning and small scanning areas.

FACTORS INFLUENCING RESOLUTION

- *Frequency*: higher frequency has a shorter wavelength, which results in better resolution, but there is decreased penetration with higher frequencies
- *Focus*: relates to "z" axis (beam width); operator can vary focus to area of interest
- *Axial resolution*: ability to discriminate between two distinct interfaces in axial (perpendicular to transducer) plane (Fig. 1-3)
- *Lateral resolution*: ability to discriminate between two distinct interfaces in lateral (horizontal) plane (Fig. 1-4)

- *Near-field/far-field resolution:*
  - Scattering degrades resolution.
  - Operator must minimize near-field scattering by adjustment of time gain compensation (TGC) or depth gain compensation (DGC).
  - Operator can optimize focus.

ARTIFACTS

- *See Figure 1-5.*
- The sonographer must be able to recognize artifacts that may simulate real echoes, including:
  - *Side lobe artifacts* created by constructions of weak off-axis wavefronts
  - *Reverberation artifacts* created at echogenic surfaces, repeated display of "pseudo" interface

TRANSDUCER DESIGN

- Some have only one focal length.
- Others have variable focus.
- Some broadband transducers give a choice of receiving frequency:
  - Lower frequencies optimize the deeper areas of interest
  - Higher frequencies optimize the closer areas of interest
- Improved resolution can be achieved by:
  - Adjustment of gain
  - Adjustment of transducer frequency (deeper structures may require lower frequency for better penetration
  - Adjustment of focus
  - Use of harmonics (Fig. 1-6): This selectively listens for harmonic (multiple of fundamental frequency), which is a weaker signal, but it provides a better signal-to-noise ratio.
  - Use of SonoCT (Fig. 1-7): This technique is available on Philips/ATL scanners and involves imaging using multiple lines of sight. Where there is image construction, true interfaces are recorded; other areas are de-emphasized as scatters.
  - Use of XRes (Fig. 1-8): This is a postprocessing algorithm that brings out certain patterns in soft-tissue structures; available on Philips/ATL scanners.

SCANNERS

- *See Figures 1-9 and 1-10.*
- Equipment ranges from large scanners equipped with a variety of probes to handheld scanners with one or two probes.

SCANNER MEMORY

- Images are stored in a digital memory, which can be characterized by its size, number of pixel elements, and depth.

DOPPLER TECHNIQUES

- Doppler techniques are used for a variety of clinical applications that involve assessment of flow dynamics.
- The technology is based on the Doppler principle that frequency shifts relate to changes in flow.
- Doppler shift is angle dependent.
- Best Doppler interrogation angle is between 30° to 60° in vessels, where the percent error of calculated velocity is less than 10%. At angles greater than 60°, major errors occur in calculated velocity.

COLOR DOPPLER SONOGRAPHY

- *See Figure 1-11.*
- Assigns a color (red or blue) to flow coursing toward or away from transducer.
- The amplitude of power Doppler relates to numbers of blood elements flowing through a vessel.

SPECTRAL ANALYSIS

- Assessment of relative velocities, as depicted by differences in transmitted and returned frequencies, can be assessed by frequency shifts or by "power" of signal.
- *Frequency shifts*: implies changes in velocity
- *Power*: relates to number of blood elements flowing
- *Impedance*: resistance to forward flow
- Impedance can be measured by several methods:

$$\text{Resistive index (R.I.)} = \frac{\text{Max. sys. vel.} - \text{dias. vel.}}{\text{Max. sys. vel.}}$$

- Advantage: relatively angle-independent values from 1.0 (highest impedance) to 0 (lowest impedance)
- Disadvantage: cannot measure if diastolic flow is reversed

$$\text{Pulsatility index (P.I.)} = \frac{\text{Max. sys.} - \text{dias. vel.}}{\text{Mean}}$$

- Advantage: takes into account more of the waveform
- Disadvantage: must measure mean velocities (done by scanner memory)

$$S/D = \frac{\text{Maximum systolic velocity}}{\text{diastolic velocity}}$$

- Advantage: simplest measure
- Disadvantage: does not take into account specifics of waveform shape
- Bioeffect considerations: sonography is considered safe and without bioeffects if used prudently.
- Intensity can be quasi-measured by:
  - *Thermal index* (TI): intensity needed to raise temperature 1°C (TI = 1.0); does not take into account cooling effect of an intact circulation
  - *Mechanical index* (MI): theoretic possibility that the intensity used could result in cavitation (production of gas bubbles) in fluid

SCANNING TECHNIQUE

- Chapters 2 and 3 provide additional details on technique.
- Sonography is highly operator dependent. It requires expert dexterity and clinical knowledge of what to look for.
- Transvaginal sonography (TVS) is used for most gynecologic applications and in early pregnancy.
- TVS should be performed using a pelvic exam table since the patient's legs can be supported and the table allows downward direction of probe (Fig. 1-12).
- Transabdominal sonography (TAS) is used for late pregnancies, and for global pelvic and abdominal imaging.
- TVS begins with the long-axis depiction of uterus; then short-axis, coronal views are obtained. The structure imaged and scan plane should be annotated on each scan.
- TAS is obtained in sagittal and transverse planes.
- A transperineal scan may be added in the second and third trimester to assess the cervix and lower uterine segment.
- Transrectal sonography can be used to guide dilation and curettage.

RECORDING AND ARCHIVING

- Images may be stored and displayed for interpretation in several ways.

PICTURE ARCHIVE COMMUNICATION SYSTEM

- *See Figure 1-13.*
- A picture archive communication system (PACS) provides electronic (film-less) display and storage.
- The advantages of PACS include digital image storage with capabilities to optimize image brightness, contrast, size, and storage and display of video loops. Other types of digital images can be displayed (CT, MR) for comparison.
- The disadvantage is that such systems are costly, and not practical for a solo practitioner.

FILM/PAPER IMAGES

- Film requires processor.
- Paper images now have acceptable latitude to be routinely used.

VIDEO

- Important for storage of heart abnormalities.
- Used for fetal condition assessment.
- Choice of VHS or super VHS (SVHS).
- SVHS has higher resolution, greater audio fidelity.

OPERATIONAL CONCERNS

- Accreditation by American Institute of Ultrasound in Medicine (AIUM) and the American College of Radiology (ACR) ensures the patient that examinations are performed to an acceptable standard of quality.
- Medicolegal concerns: be cognizant of the standards that have been established for routine obstetric and gynecologic ultrasound.

KEY FUNDAMENTAL CONCEPTS

- Be aware of the advantages and limitations of each type of transvaginal probe. Select the one that will optimize image quality and result in the most complete examination.
- Documentation of area of structure imaged and plane of section is important.
- Diagnostic sonography used for gynecology and obstetric applications has no known detrimental bioeffects.
- Doppler techniques depict physiologic parameters and vascularity.
- The standards for gynecologic and obstetric sonography specify what should be included in each sonographic study. These are included in Appendix 1 and Appendix 2 at the end of the book. Sonographers should be familiar with the contents of these standards and follow the guidelines for each study they perform and interpret.

REFERENCES

O'Brien WD Jr, Siddiqi TA. Obstetric sonography: the output display standard and ultrasound bioeffects. In: Fleischer AC, Manning F, Jeanty P, Romero R, eds. *Sonography in Obstetrics and Gynecology: Principles and Practice*, ed 6. New York: McGraw-Hill, 2001:29.

Price RR, Fleischer AC, Abuhamad AZ. Sonographic instrumentation and operational concerns. In: Fleischer AC, Manning F, Jeanty P, Romero R, eds. *Sonography in Obstetrics and Gynecology: Principles and Practice*, ed 6. New York: McGraw-Hill, 2001:1.

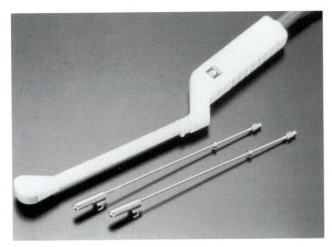

A

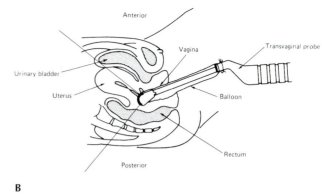

B

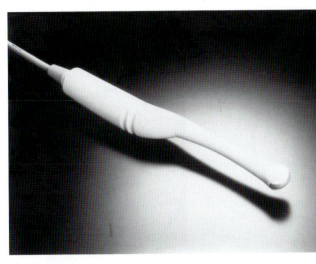

C

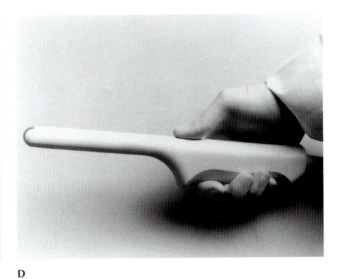

D

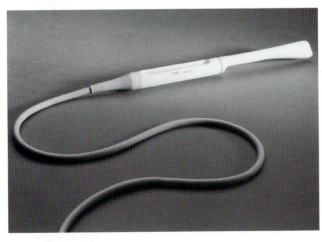

E

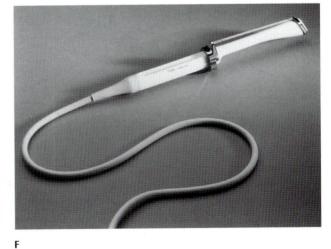

F

FIGURE 1-1 (A) Curved linear array transvaginal probe with needle guide attachments. **(B)** Diagram of curved linear array transvaginal probe, illustrating approximate field of view. (*Courtesy of Toshiba, Inc.*) **(C)** "Tightly" curved transvaginal probe that uses 200 subelements with a central frequency of 6 MHz. (*Courtesy of Toshiba America US, Inc.*) **(D)** ATL convex transvaginal probe that operates at 5-9 MHz. (*Courtesy of ATL, Inc.*) **(E)** Phased array transvaginal probe with a tilted "footprint." This probe allows imaging with selectable frequencies of 5.0, 6.5, or 7.5 MHz. (*Courtesy of Acuson, Inc.*) **(F)** Same probe as in **E** with needle guide attached. (*Courtesy of Acuson, Inc.*)

FIGURE 1-2 (A) Traditional linear sequenced arrays (left) produce rectangular fields of view and use both transmit and receive array focusing. Phased linear arrays (right) are steered to produce a sector-shaped field of view and also to use both transmit and receive focusing. **(B)** Radial or convex linear arrays provide increased field of view with depth without electronic scanning, thus reducing grating-lobe artifacts that accompany traditional phased arrays when large steering angles are used.

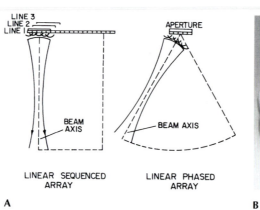

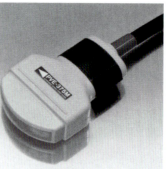

A

B

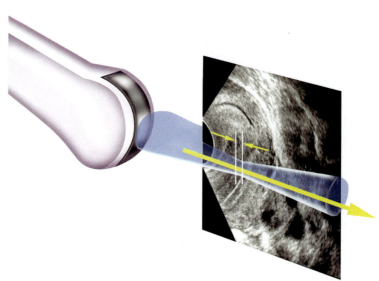

FIGURE 1-3 Axial resolution, the ability to depict interfaces in the direction of the beam path.

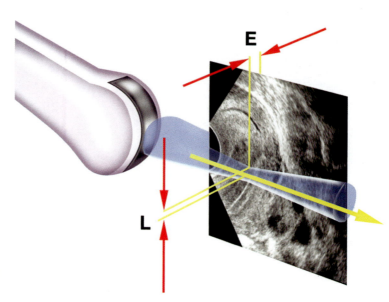

FIGURE 1-4 Lateral (L) resolution and elevational resolution (E) within the beam.

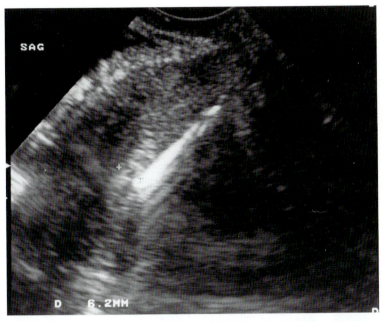

A

FIGURE 1-5 Artifacts. **(A)** Multiple reverberation artifacts arising from an intrauterine contraceptive device. *(Figure continued.)*

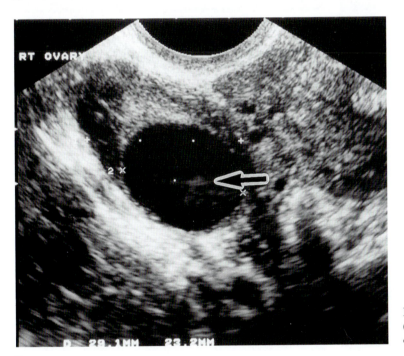

B

FIGURE 1-5 *(continued)* **(B)** A side lobe artifact (*arrow*) is producing spurious echoes within a simple ovarian cyst in the right ovary.

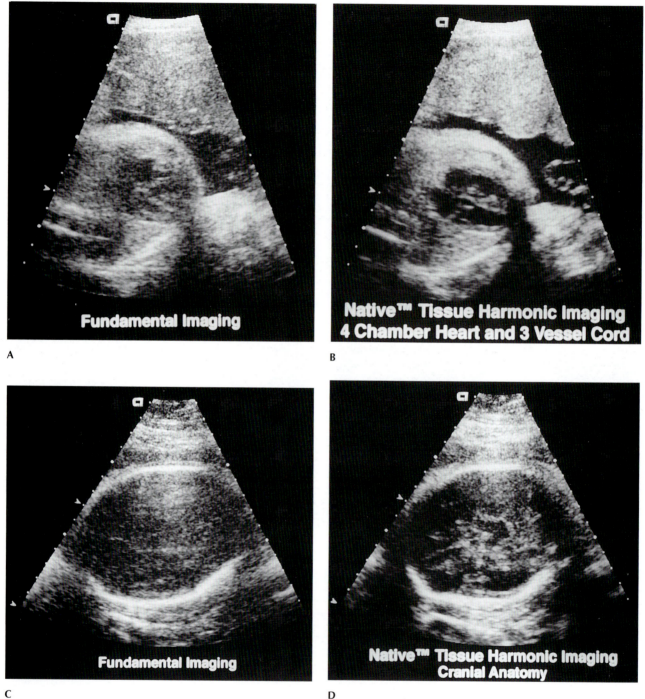

A

B

C

D

FIGURE 1-6 Harmonic imaging applications in obstetrics and gynecology. **(A)** Fundamental transverse sonogram of the fetal chest at 29 weeks of gestation in a difficult-to-image patient with multiple abdominal scarring from prior surgeries. The presence of an anterior placenta and decreased amniotic fluid volume adds to the difficulty of this exam. In **A**, the sonographer is attempting to obtain a four-chamber view of the fetal heart. As seen, imaging is suboptimal and a four-chamber view of the fetal heart could not be obtained. **(B)** Images of the same patient shown in **A** in the same plane using Native Tissue Harmonic Imaging (*Courtesy of Acuson, Inc.*). Now the four-chamber view is clearly imaged. A three-vessel transverse segment of the umbilical cord is also imaged within the amniotic fluid. **(C)** Fundamental transverse sonogram of the fetal head at 34 weeks of gestation in a difficult-to-image patient with severe oligohydramnios. In this case, the sonographer is attempting to image fetal intracranial anatomy, but imaging is suboptimal. **(D)** Images of the same patient in the same place as in **C** using Native Tissue Harmonic Imaging. The interhemispheric fissure, thalamus, and insula are now clearly seen. *(Figure continued.)*

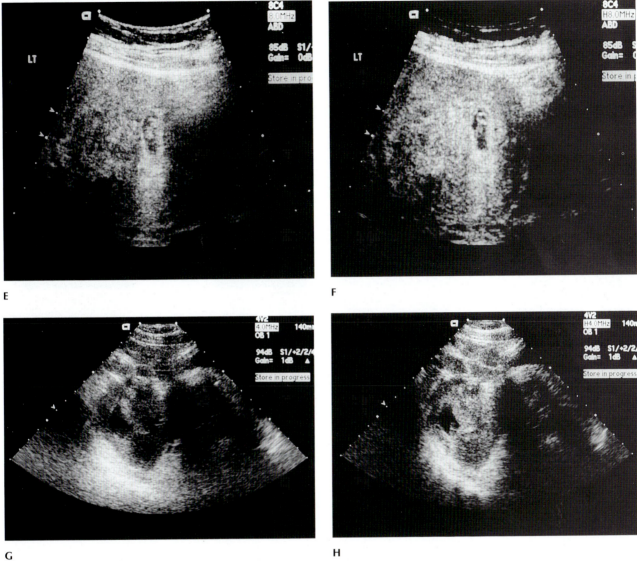

E

F

G

H

FIGURE 1-6 *(continued)* **(E)** Transabdominal fundamental sonogram of an enlarged uterus in a patient presenting to the emergency room with abdominal pain and positive pregnancy test. Endovaginal sonography showed an enlarged uterus with a large fibroid. Due to the size of the uterus, the endometrial cavity could not be assessed, and so an intrauterine pregnancy could not be confirmed by endovaginal scanning. On fundamental transabdominal sonography, a suspicion of an intrauterine gestation is present; however, a fetal pole and a yolk sac could not be confirmed. **(F)** Same patient as in **E**, using Native Tissue Harmonic Imaging. Note the clear delineation of a yolk sac within the gestation, thus confirming an intrauterine pregnancy. **(G)** Transabdominal fundamental sonogram of a difficult-to-image patient referred with a positive pregnancy test. A fetal pole could not be documented by fundamental imaging. **(H)** Same patient as in **G**, using Native Tissue Harmonic Imaging. A fetal pole is clearly seen within a gestation sac, and the patient was thus reassured. *(Courtesy of Alfred Abuhamad, M.D.)*

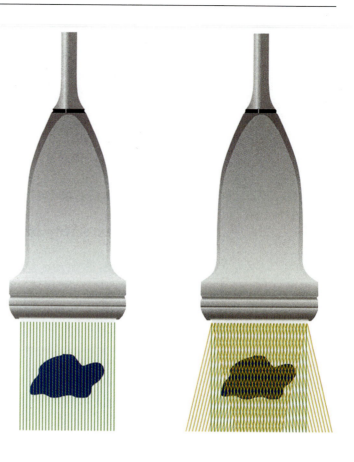

FIGURE 1-7 SonoCT utilizes multiple lines of sight, optimizing signal-to-noise ratio.

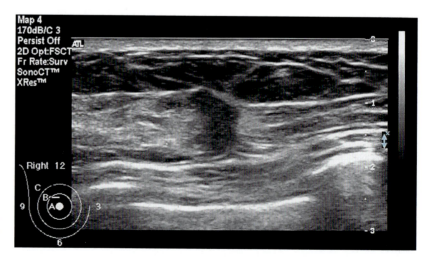

FIGURE 1-8 XRes technology enhances the depiction of soft tissue detail, such as this breast mass relative to surrounding fat.

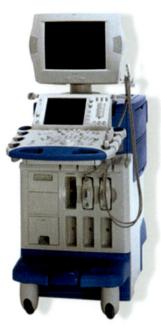

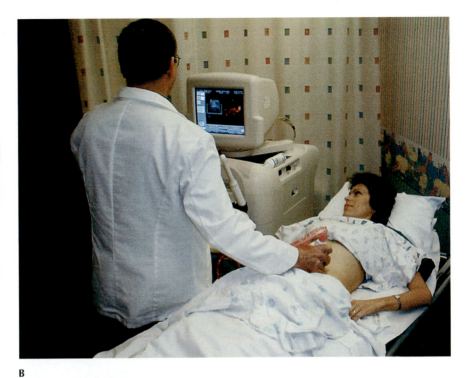

A

B

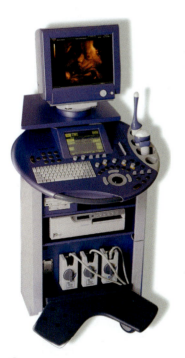

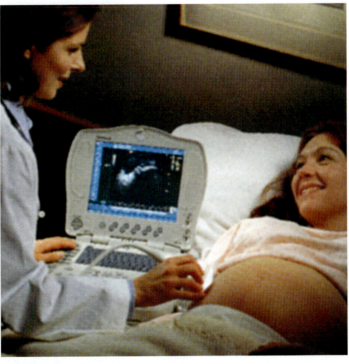

C

D

FIGURE 1-9 (A) Toshiba's Aplio scanner is capable of all types of scanning, including transabdominal, transvaginal, and transrectal probes. (*Courtesy of Toshiba America Medical Systems, Inc.*) **(B)** Philips/ATL 4000 being used to scan a patient's abdomen. (*Courtesy of Phil Williams, R.D.M.S., and Galina Bell, M.D.*) **(C)** G.E.'s Voluson 730 is capable of all type of scanning, including "4D." (*Courtesy of G.E. Medical Systems, Inc.*) **(D)** G.E.'s Logic Book Scanner is the size of a laptop computer. (*Courtesy of G.E. Medical Systems, Inc.*)

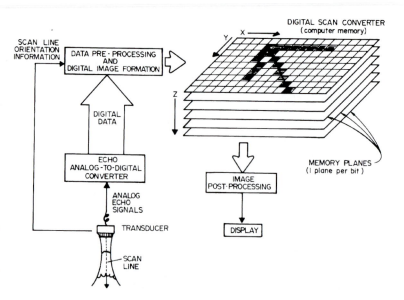

FIGURE 1-10 Block diagram of a digital ultrasound system. Echo signals detected by the transducer are digitized and then stored in computer memory (digital scan converter), which is then read out to a video monitor.

FIGURE 1-11 Principles of color Doppler sonography (CDS). **(A)** Diagram showing Doppler equation to calculate flow velocity. The change in emitted (f_0) and returned (f_r) frequency (Δf) is related to the angle of insonation ($\cos\theta$). (*Courtesy of W. Charboneau, M.D.*) **(B)** Methods to measure flow from Doppler waveform. *(Figure continued.)*

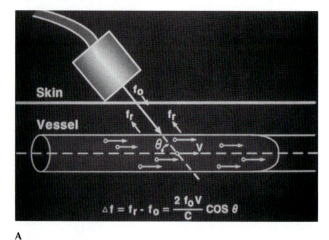

$$\Delta f = f_r - f_0 = \frac{2 f_0 V}{C} \cos\theta$$

A

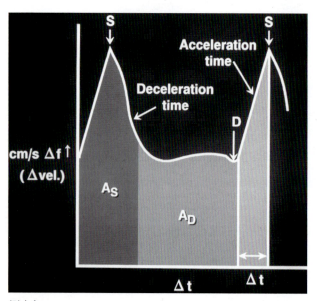

(B) left

Systolic/Diastolic	=	S/D
Resistive Index (R.I.)	=	$\dfrac{S\text{-}D}{S}$
Pulsatility Index (P.I.)	=	$\dfrac{S\text{-}D}{mean}$
Acceleration to peak (Acc)	=	$\dfrac{vel.\ (max) - vel\ (min)}{t\ (beginning\ of\ systolic\ to\ max) - t\ (time\ to\ peak\ systole)}$
Perfusion Index (Per I)	=	$\dfrac{\int\ Area\ under\ curve\ during\ systole}{\int\ Area\ under\ curve\ during\ diastole}$
Deceleration time (Dec)	=	$\dfrac{\Delta v}{\Delta t}$ (First derivative decrease in diastole/time)
Impedance Index (IMI)	=	$\dfrac{S\ mean}{D^2}$

(B) right

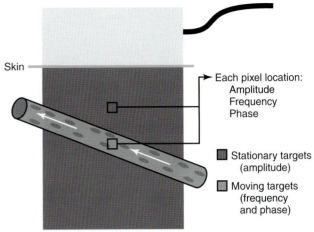

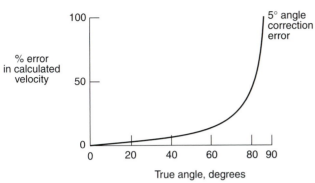

C

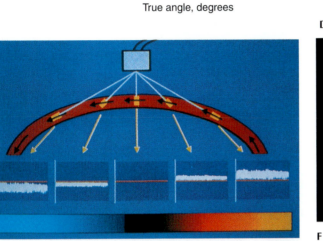

E

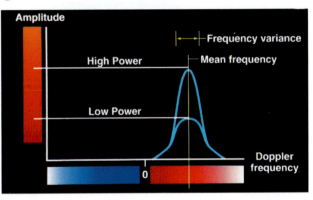

F

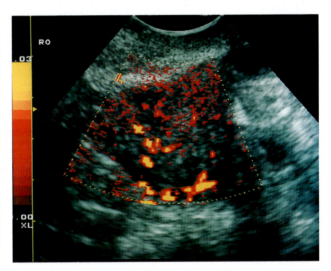

G

H

FIGURE 1-11 *(continued)* **(C)** Graph depicting percentage of error relative to the angle of insonation. There is a minimal error in calculated velocity up to 60 degrees. **(D)** Diagram of the components of the color Doppler sonogram showing flow information obtained from moving targets recorded over a gray-scale depiction of interfaces. **(E)** Diagram showing color assignment of flow and waveform display. The waveform is depicted above the baseline if it is going toward the transducer, below if away. It is depicted in red if moving toward the transducer or blue if it is moving away. Doppler signals are not readily obtained perpendicular to the transducer and are shown in black. **(F)** Relationship between frequency and amplitude or power CDS. Frequency-based CDS is based on differences in transmitted and received frequencies. The flow is coded with red if the flow is toward the transducer, with blue if it is away. Frequency CDS reflects changes in velocity as they relate to flow. Amplitude CDS reflects the number of blood elements or power flowing within a field of view. The Doppler shifts are coded in shades of orange. **(G)** Directional amplitude color Doppler sonography displays directional information (red = toward, blue = away) superimposed on flow. **(H)** Amplitude CDS of the right ovary shown in **G** shows flow around a corpus luteum and is more sensitive to flow but does not discriminate its directional flow.

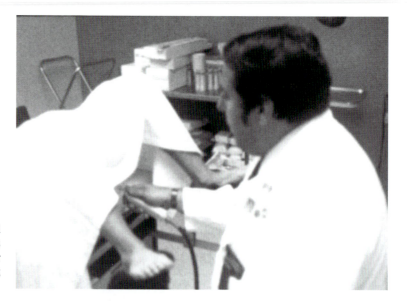

FIGURE 1-12 Transvaginal sonography performed with the patient on a pelvic exam table with her legs supported. The exam table also allows the transducer handle to be directed downward for optimal imaging of an anteflexed uterus.

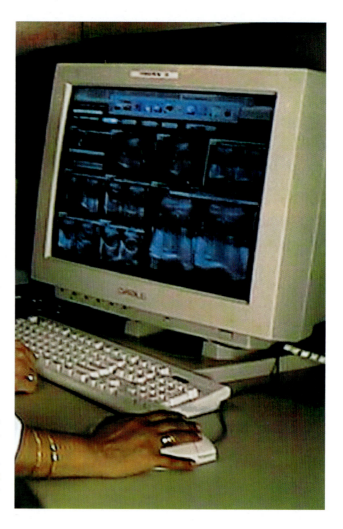

FIGURE 1-13 Ultrasound PACS. Several sonographic images are displayed on the monitor and stored electronically. The digital storage process allows manipulation and optimization of the images. Several scanners can be hooked up to this display module. The systems greatly enhance sonographer productivity and throughput because there is no need to take, process, or store films. (*Courtesy of ALI, Inc.*)

2 NORMAL PELVIC ANATOMY

OVERVIEW

- Transabdominal sonography (TAS) provides a global overview of the uterus and ovaries.
- Transvaginal sonography (TVS) provides a detailed depiction of the uterus, endometrium, and ovaries.
- The optimal scan plane is empirically determined by sonographer during exam.
- Sonographer can use the probe to displace uterus from ovary and/or move bowel loops away from area of interest, and coax the uterus and/or ovary (by applying gentle pressure) into optimal position for TVS.
- Use uterus as central landmark.
- Use internal iliac vein as landmark for ovarian "fossa" to locate the usual position of the ovary.

UTERUS

- *See Figures 2-1 through 2-7.*
- Size and shape are related to whether patient is pre- or post-pubertal, nulliparous or multiparous, and/or pre-, peri-, or postmenopausal:
  - *Normal size* (adult): 6 to 8 cm in length (long axis) and 3 to 5 cm in the transverse and anterioposterior (short axis) dimension
  - *Pre-pubertal*: comprised mostly of cervix, small corpus/fundus
  - *Post-pubertal*: corpus, fundus enlarges
  - *Nulliparous*: corpus, fundus larger than cervix
  - *Multiparous*: enlarged over nulliparous, more "flexible"; can go from anteflexed when scanned with a distended bladder to retroflexed when scanned on TVS
  - *Postmenopausal*: small compared to perimenopausal; late postmenopausal is similar in size to pre-pubertal
- Varies in location, "rotation" (ante- versus retroflexed versus neutral position; see Fig. 2-4).
- Arterial supply comes from the hypogastric artery (internal iliac artery), and then branches into ascending and descending (cervical) branches.
- Veins roughly parallel arteries.

- Between the outer and the middle layers of myometrium, the arcuate vessels extend in a spokewheel fashion to give off radial and then spiral branches in the endometrium.
- Three myometrial layers:
  - *Inner*: relatively hypoechoic due to arrangement of muscle fibers; assists in endometrial peristalisis
  - *Middle*: main muscle layer, arranged in spiral configuration
  - *Outer*: contiguous with tubal musculature
- Arcuate vessels are positioned at the boundary between the outer and middle myometrial layers.

ENDOMETRIUM

- *See Figures 2-8 through 2-11.*
- Consists of a basal layer (not shed) and a functional layer (which sloughs, thickens, and is shed each month).
- Postmenopausal endometrium consists mostly of the basal layer.
- In women of childbearing age (not suppressed), the endometrium changes in texture and thickness according to the menstrual cycle:
  - Menstrual days 0–5: menstrual phase irregular; can appear as a sheath of sloughed tissue
  - Days 5–13: follicular or proliferative phase; homogenous, mildly echogenic
  - Days 13–15: peri-ovulatory phase; can see multi-layered appearance consisting of median echogenic interface arising from the mucous functionalis layer, which is relatively hypoechoic; then the basal layer, which is mildly echogenic
  - Days 15–26: luteal or secretory phase; thickest and most echogenic
  - Days 20–28: ischemic phase; similar to luteal phase
- Basal veins are parallel to basal endometrium.
- Spiral vessels can be seen within the endometrium in the luteal phase.
- The contraction of the inner layer of the myometrium results in endometrial "peristalsis." This is vital in the transport of sperm into the fundal region and for the sloughing of endometrium from fundus to cervix during menses. It can best be seen when recorded on videotape and played at twice normal speed.

OVARIES

- Ovaries vary in size depending on age and menopausal status. Normal size is approximately 3 × 2 × 2 cm.
- Almond-shaped
- Contain follicles in women of childbearing age
- Follicles are less than 10 mm when immature; 10 to 15 mm at intermediate maturity; and 18 to 25 mm when mature.
- Corpora lutea: thick wall, vascular "ring"
- The main arterial supply of the uterus and ovaries arises from the aorta through the infundibulopelvic ligament; other blood supply is from the adnexal branch of the uterine artery (Fig. 2-12).
- There is high-impedance arterial flow except around the mature follicle/corpora lutea, where low-impedance, high-diastolic flow can be seen.

OTHER STRUCTURES

- *See Figure 2-13.*
- The tube is usually not seen, except when dilated or when there is fluid on either side of it. The tube appears as a tortuous structure coursing from the uterus and continuing to the ovary, typically in a cul-de-sac.

- Bowel is usually not seen unless it is inflamed or neoplastic; it usually can be compressed.
- Distended parauterine/ovarian veins are usually seen more on the left than the right.

KEY FUNDAMENTAL CONCEPTS

- The uterus serves as the landmark for imaging the adnexa.
- Uterine and ovarian size vary with age.
- The sonographic appearance of the endometrium varies during the normal menstrual cycle and can be related to developmental stage—follicular, periovulatory, and luteal.
- Ovaries are readily depicted with TVS due to the follicles/corpora lutea.

REFERENCES

Fleischer AC, Kepple DM. Normal pelvic anatomy as depicted with transvaginal sonography. In: Fleischer AC, Manning F, Jeanty P, Romero R, eds. *Sonography in Obstetrics and Gynecology: Principles and Practice*, ed. 6. New York: McGraw-Hill, 2001:49.

Pavlik EJ, DePriest PD, Gallion HH, et al. Ovarian volume related to age. *Gynecol Oncol.* 2000;77:410.

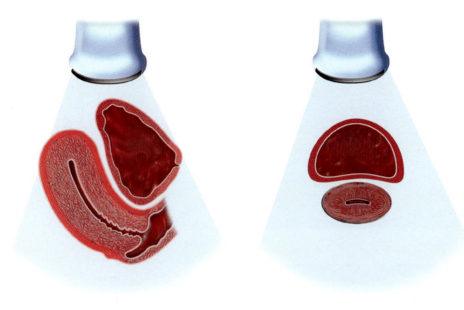

Long Axis   Short Axis

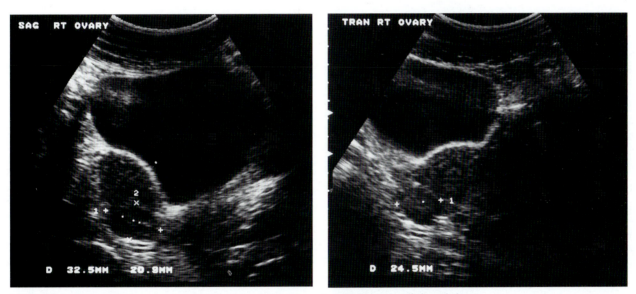

FIGURE 2-1 Scanning planes used with transabdominal sonography (TAS) in long (*left*) and short (*right*) axis with accompanying typical sonograms showing uterus and right ovary in sagittal plane and right ovary and uterus in transverse plane. By convention, the left of the image depicts the cephalic or superior aspect of the patient whereas the right of the patient is depicted on the left of the image of the transverse scans.

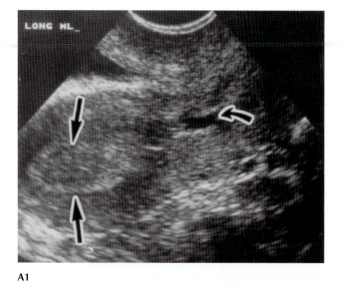

A1

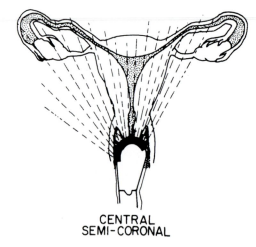

CENTRAL
SEMI-CORONAL

A2

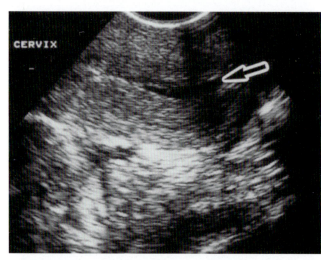

B1

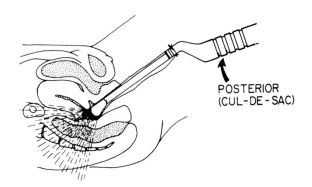

POSTERIOR
(CUL-DE-SAC)

B2

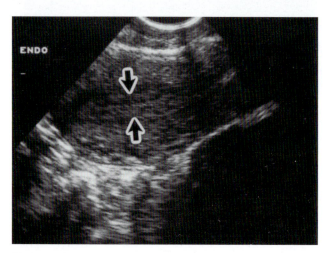

C1

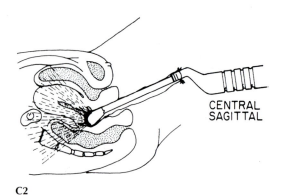

CENTRAL
SAGITTAL

C2

FIGURE 2-2 Uterus, endometrium, and cervix. Drawings depict plane of section. **(A)** Long axis of uterus in semicoronal plane showing the endometrium (*arrows*) and the cervix. There is a small amount of fluid (*curved arrow*) within the endocervical canal. **(B)** Same patient after withdrawing the probe into the mid-vagina. The endocervical canal with its fluid mucus (*arrow*) is clearly seen. **(C)** Long axis of endometrium (*arrowheads*) during the proliferative phase. It is relatively hypo-echoic at this state. *(Figure continued.)*

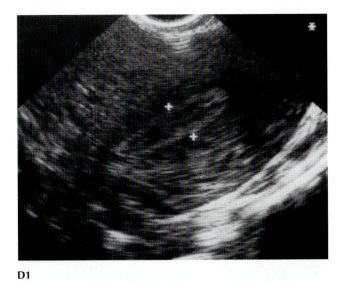

D1

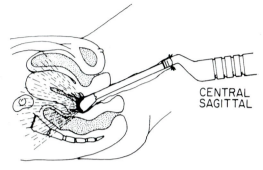

D2

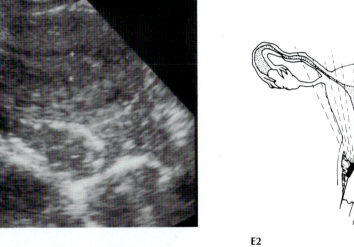

E1

E2

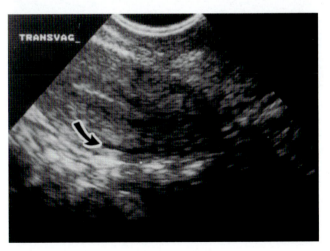

F1

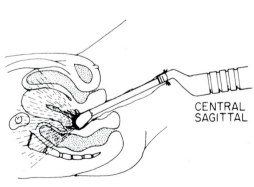

F2

FIGURE 2-2 *(continued)* **(D)** Long axis of the endometrium during the periovulatory phase showing hypoechoic inner layer. The multilayered endometrium is clearly seen between the cursors. **(E)** Long axis of endometrium *(between cursors)* in secretory phase, appearing as echogenic tissue (reversed orientation with uterine fundus to right of image). **(F)** Oblique image showing arcuate veins *(arrow)* within outer myometrium. *(Figure continued.)*

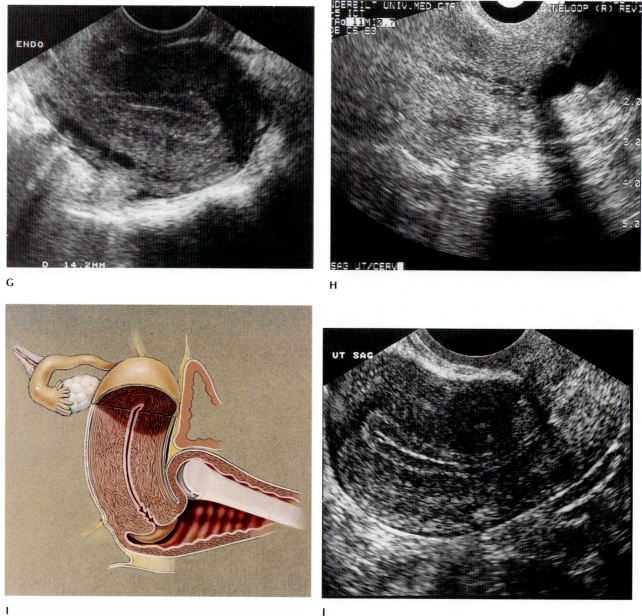

FIGURE 2-2 *(continued)* **(G)** TVS of retroflexed uterus with distended arcuate veins. The endometrium *(between cursors)* shows a typical secretory phase pattern. **(H)** TVS showing two large cervical inclusion cysts. **(I)** Transducer/probe motion to enhance depiction of the uterus and endometrium in an anteflexed uterus. The probe is placed in the anterior vaginal fornix and directed anteriorly. **(J)** Complete delineation of the multilayered endometrium in long axis. *(Figure continued.)*

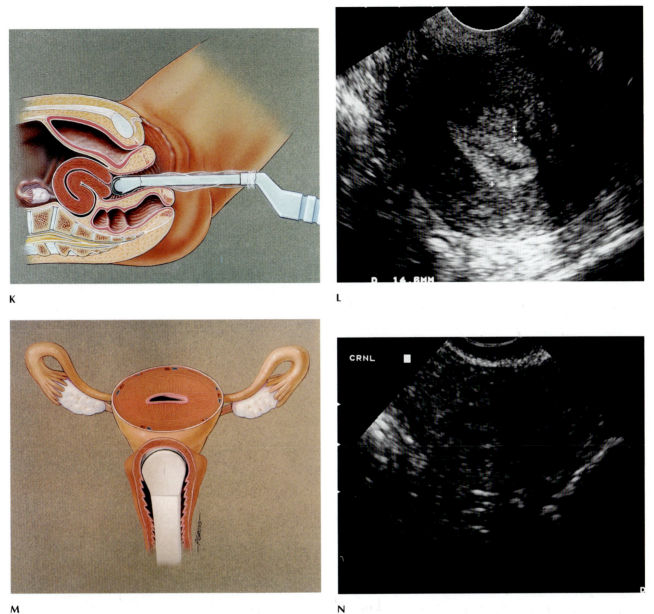

K

L

M

N

FIGURE 2-2 *(continued)* **(K)** Transducer probe showing direction of probe used to enhance depiction of a retroflexed uterus. **(L)** Corresponding TVS of drawing shown in **K** showing retroflexed uterus with secretory phase endometrium (between cursors). **(M)** Diagram showing short-axis image of endometrium. **(N)** Corresponding TVS of image plane in **M** showing short-axis view of the endometrium with surrounding hypoechoic inner myometrium.

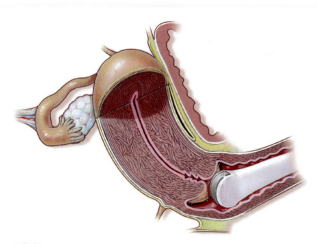

A (left)

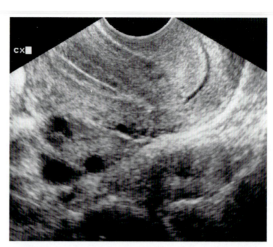

A (right)

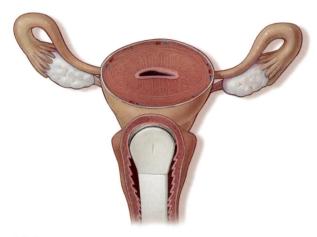

B (left)

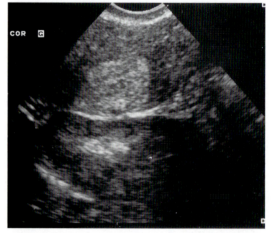

B (right)

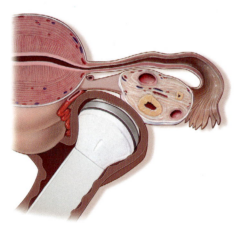

C (left)

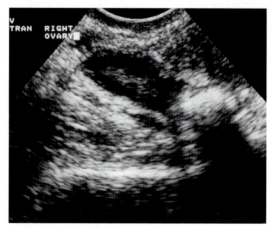

C (right)

FIGURE 2-3 Scanning planes used with transvaginal sonography (TVS). **(A)** Midline sagittal view (*left*) depicting uterus is long axis with accompanying transvaginal sonogram. The sagittal image (*right*) is oriented with anterior or superior aspect of the patient to left of image. **(B)** Short-axis view of uterus (*left*) with an accompanying transvaginal sonogram (*right*) showing increased through transmission of the luteal phase endometrium. **(C)** Adnexal view of ovary (*left*) with accompanying transvaginal sonogram (*right*) in semiaxial or transverse plane; the patient's right is displayed on the left.

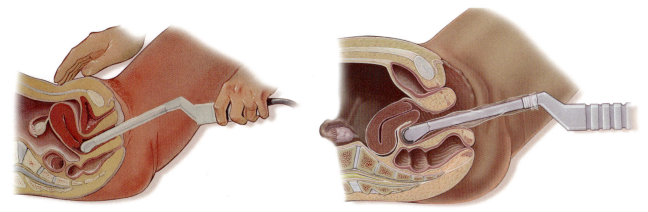

FIGURE 2-4 Ante- (*left*) versus retro- (*right*) flexed uterus as depicted by TVS. The sonographer must direct the probe anteriorly for optimal depiction of the anteflexed uterus, whereas the retroflexed uterus lies directly in the scan plane.

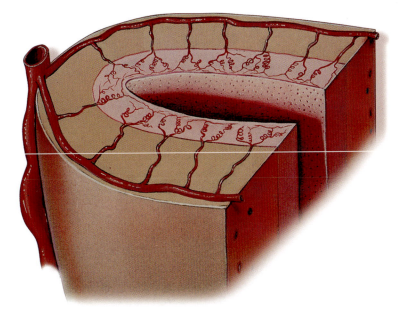

FIGURE 2-5 Arterial vascularity of the uterus. The main uterine artery branches from the hypogastric artery (internal iliac artery) and courses along the lateral edges of the uterus, branching off into the arcuates. The radial arteries then course towards the endometrium, branching into the basal and spiral arteries within the endometrium.

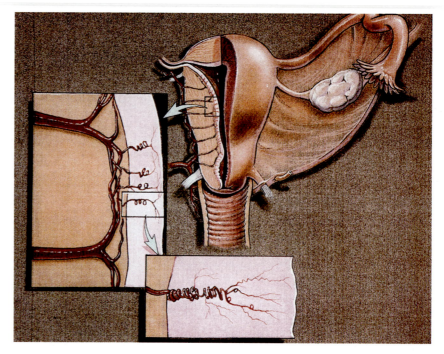

FIGURE 2-6 Diagram of the uterine arterial tree. The arcuate arterioles branch into radial arteries that course across the myometrium ending in the spiral arteries within the endometrium.

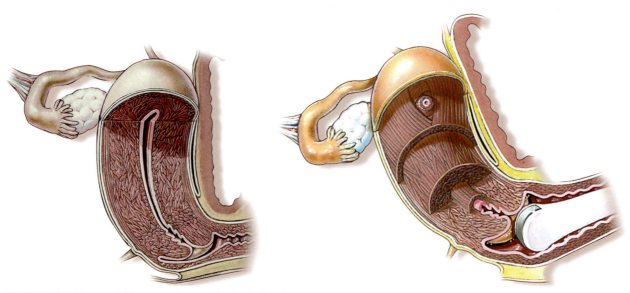

FIGURE 2-7 Myometrial layers as depicted by TVS (*left* shows midline; *right* shows layers). The innermost layer of myometrium is hypoechoic and provides endometrial peristalsis (in light pink). The middle layer is the thickest and arranged in a spiral fashion (shown as muscle bundles). The outermost layer extends from the arcuate vessels to the serosa and is contiguous with the musculature of the tube.

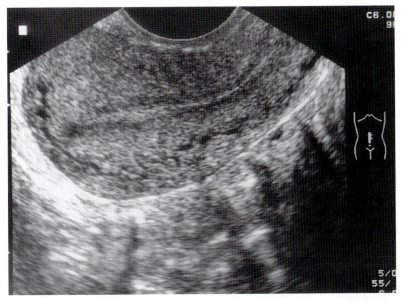

A

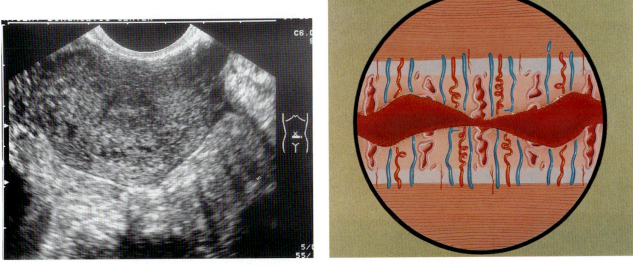

B (left)   **B** (right)

FIGURE 2-8 Normal endometrium as depicted by TVS. Long **(A)** and short **(B)** axes of early pro-liferative endometrium. Transvaginal sonograms (*left*) and accompanying diagram show micro-scopic anatomy of the endometrium (*right*). (*Diagram by Paul Gross, M.S.*) (*Figure continued.*)

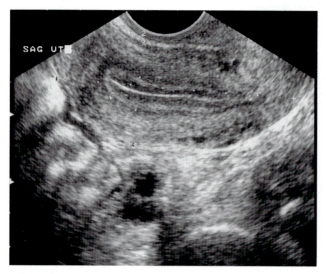

C (left)

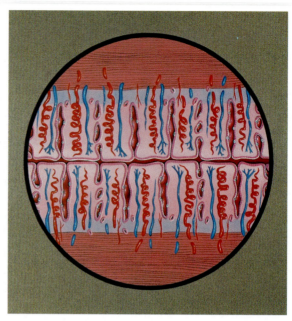

C (right)

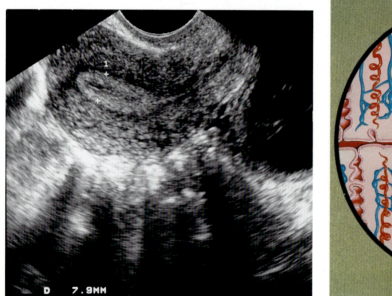

D (left)

D (right)

FIGURE 2-8 *(continued)* **(C)** Long axis of endometrium in midcycle *(left)*. A multilayered appearance is seen with the outer echogenic interface representing basalis, the inner layer functionalis, and the median echo from refluxed mucus. Diagram of corresponding microscopic anatomy *(right)*. The glandular elements and stroma enlarge, whereas the basal layer (light blue) remains constant. **(D)** Luteal phase endometrium appearing as thick (8 mm), regular, and echogenic *(left)*. Diagram showing thickened stroma and distended glands *(right)*. *(Figure continued.)*

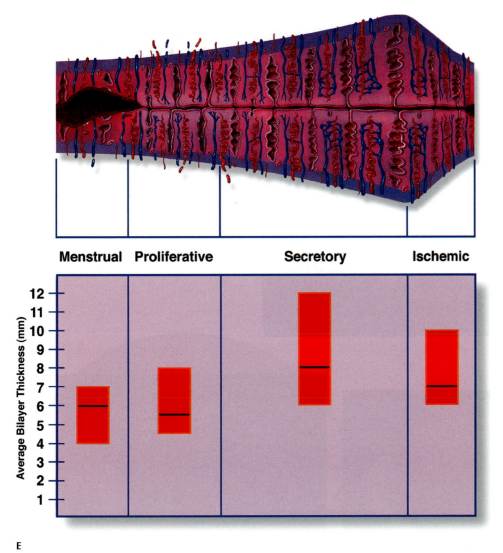

| Menstrual | Proliferative | Secretory | Ischemic |

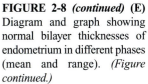

FIGURE 2-8 *(continued)* **(E)** Diagram and graph showing normal bilayer thicknesses of endometrium in different phases (mean and range). *(Figure continued.)*

E

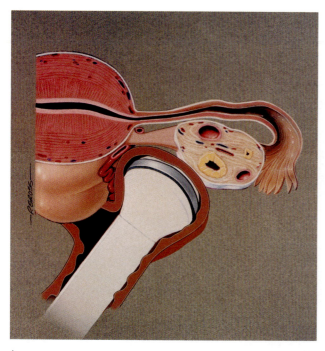

A

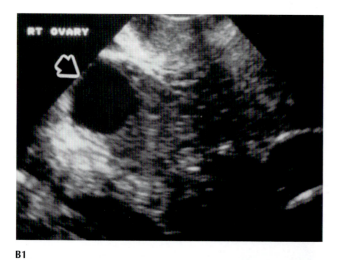

B1

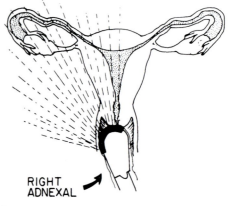

RIGHT
ADNEXAL

B2

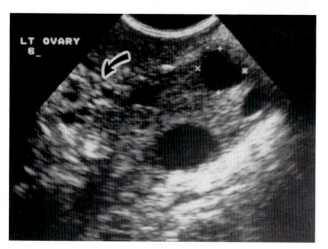

C1

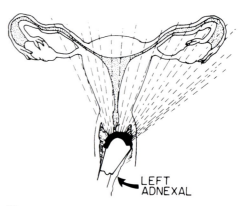

LEFT
ADNEXAL

C2

FIGURE 2-11 (A) Transducer probe direction for depiction of the ovary and tube. **(B)** Right ovary containing a mature follicle (*arrow*) in a spontaneous cycle. **(C)** Left ovary containing fresh corpus luteum (*cursors*). The wall is thick and irregular secondary to luteinization. Some pericervical vessels (*curved arrow*) are also seen. *(Figure continued.)*

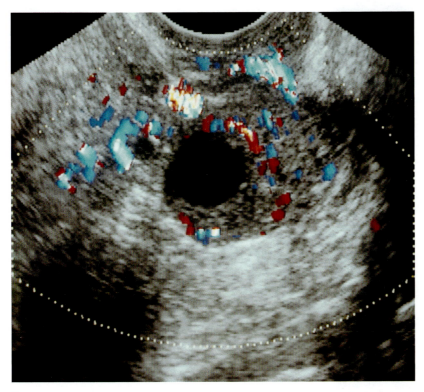

D

FIGURE 2-11 *(continued)* **(D)** Transvaginal color Doppler sonogram of a mature follicle showing blood flow within the ovary.

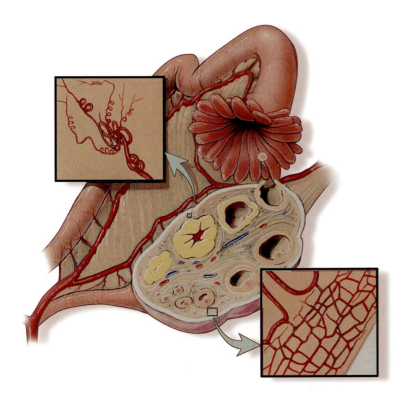

FIGURE 2-12 Ovarian vasculature. The ovary has a dual blood supply, mainly off the aorta through the ovarian artery and the adenexal branch of the uterine artery. Then several capsular vessels course into the ovary. Within the ovary, the arterial and venous flow depends on the presence of a functioning corpus luteum. When there is a functioning corpus luteum, a vascular wreath of vessels with low impedance flow can be detected on CDS. The ovarian veins roughly parallel the arteries and join to form the gonadal veins, which drain into the left renal vein in the left and the inferior vena cana on the right.

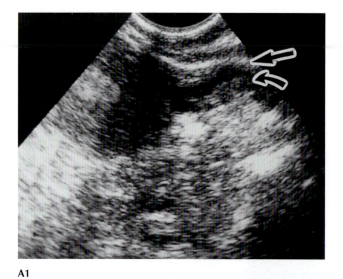

A1

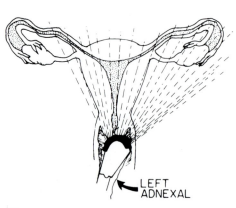

A2

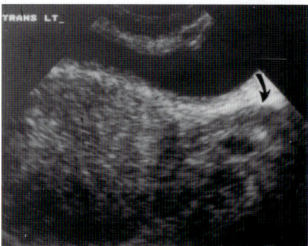

B1

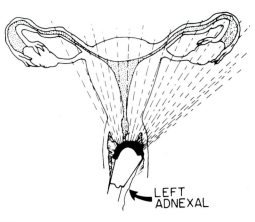

B2

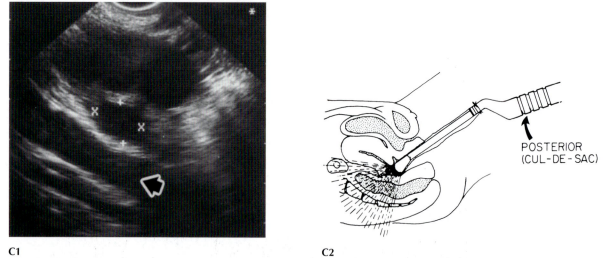

C1   C2

FIGURE 2-13 Other pelvic structures. Drawings depict plane of section. **(A)** Normal left tube (*curved arrow*) arising from cornual area adjacent to the uterine attachment of the round ligament (*straight arrow*). **(B)** Normal left uterine tube (*curved arrow*) extending from left uterine corpus. **(C)** Internal iliac vein (*arrow*) and artery in long axis adjacent to a follicle-containing ovary. *(Figure continued.)*

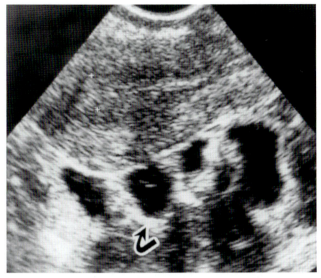

D1

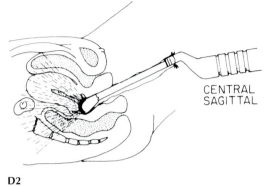

CENTRAL
SAGITTAL

D2

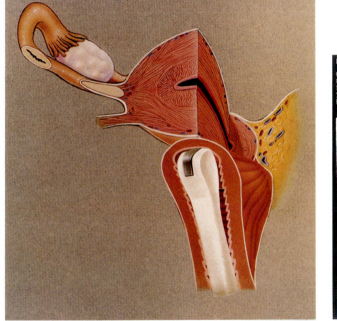

E

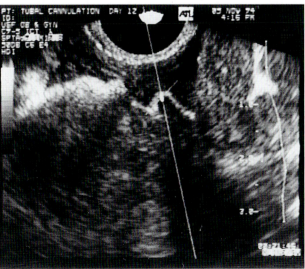

F

FIGURE 2-13 *(continued)* **(D)** Fluid-filled small bowel *(curved arrow)* surrounded by intraperitoneal fluid. **(E)** To evaluate the tube, one begins by identifying the area of the tubal ostia. The endometrium invaginates into the uterine cornua, particularly when it is thick and echogenic in the luteal phase. **(F)** TVS showing area of tube. The actual lumen and tube cannot be routinely depicted on TVS without the use of saline or contrast. With contrast injection, the tortuous course of the tube is depicted. *(Courtesy of A. Parsons, M.D.)*

3 UTERINE DISORDERS

OVERVIEW

- Sonography has an important role in the identification of fibroids and the evaluation of their size and location.
- Fibroids (leiomyomas, also known as myomas) are uterine tumors that consist of smooth muscle and connective tissue.
- They are commonly associated with abnormal bleeding, pain, infertility, and pressure symptoms involving the urinary bladder or bowel.
- Sonography is also useful in evaluation of uterine malformations; 3D sonography (3D US) is particularly helpful.
- Adenomyosis is a common cause of pelvic pain and can be identified using transvaginal sonography (TVS).

SCANNING TECHNIQUE

- *See Figures 3-1 and 3-2.*
- Transabdominal sonography (TAS) performed with a fully distended bladder provides an excellent overview of uterine size, flexion, and symmetry.
- TVS best depicts irregularities within the myometrium or malformations of the uterus.
- TVS should first depict long axis of uterus with several images followed by short-axis views and if necessary "down the barrel" or semi-coronal views.
- Rotation of the probe relative to the uterus may result in an inaccurate depiction of uterine size, shape, and symmetry.
- To minimize this, orient images of uterus relative to its central long axis and short axis.

NORMAL

- *See Figures 3-3 through 3-5.*
- Uterine size and shape (configuration) vary.

- Uterine size is not as clinically important as its shape and texture.
- Normal uterine size of an adult woman is approximately 6 to 8 cm in length, and 3 to 5 cm in the anterioposterior and transverse dimensions.
- *Configuration* refers to the relative proportions of cervix, corpus, and fundus:
  - An oblong shape is normal.
  - A T-shaped uterus is associated with maternal diethylstilbesterol (DES) exposure.
  - A pre-pubertal uterus is comprised mostly of cervix.
  - A post-pubertal uterus shows an enlargement of corpus and fundus relative to pre-pubertal proportions.
  - A multiparous is larger than a nulliparous uterus.
  - A postmenopausal uterus is smaller, approximately the same size as the post-pubertal uterus.

FLEXION

- *Anteflexed*: fundus is anteriorly directed relative to cervix
- *Retroflexed*: fundus is posteriorly directed relative to cervix
- *Neutral position*: neither ante- or retroflexed; difficult to image with TVS
- TVS usually depicts the uterus in a "down the barrel" view.
- Gentle fundal pressure may help establish when the probe is in a more optimal scan plane.

MALFORMATIONS AND ACQUIRED ABNORMALITIES

- *See Figures 3-6 and 3-7.*
- *Bicornuate*: two separate endometrial lumina with a fundal cleft
- *Septated*: two separate endometrial lumina with no fundal cleft
- A septated uterus is more commonly associated with fertility problems because the conceptus may have difficulty implanting on the septum.

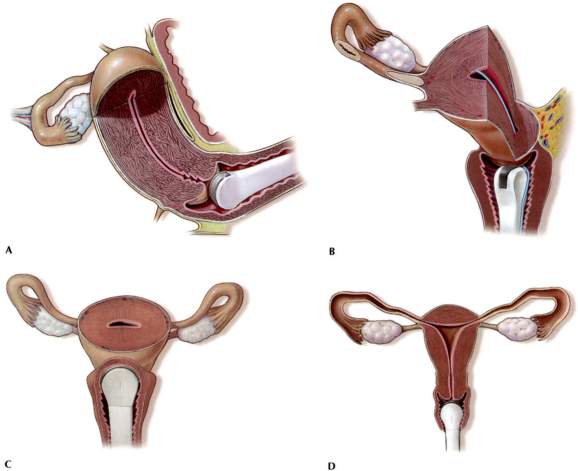

A   B

C   D

FIGURE 3-2 Scan planes used for TVS of the uterus. **(A)** First, the long axis of the uterus is imaged. **(B)** The probe is angled toward the right, then the left, cornu in the semi-sagittal plane. A sonohysterography catheter is shown in its long axis. **(C)** Next, the probe is rotated to image the uterus in short axis, sweeping from fundus to cervix. **(D)** Additional views can be obtained by directing the probe in a semi-coronal plane. In this plane, the transverse endometrial thickness is obtained.

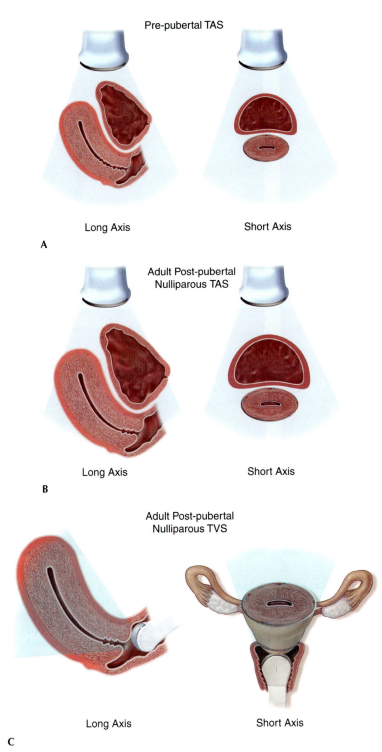

Pre-pubertal TAS

Long Axis   Short Axis

A

Adult Post-pubertal
Nulliparous TAS

Long Axis   Short Axis

B

Adult Post-pubertal
Nulliparous TVS

Long Axis   Short Axis

C

FIGURE 3-3 Normal size and configuration of the uterus in the long and short axes. **(A)** TAS of pre-pubertal uterus. Note the size of the cervix relative to the corpus and fundus. **(B)** TAS of adult post-pubertal, nulliparous uterus. The corpus and fundus have enlarged when compared to prepubertal size. **(C)** TVS of adult post-pubertal, nulliparous uterus. *(Figure continued.)*

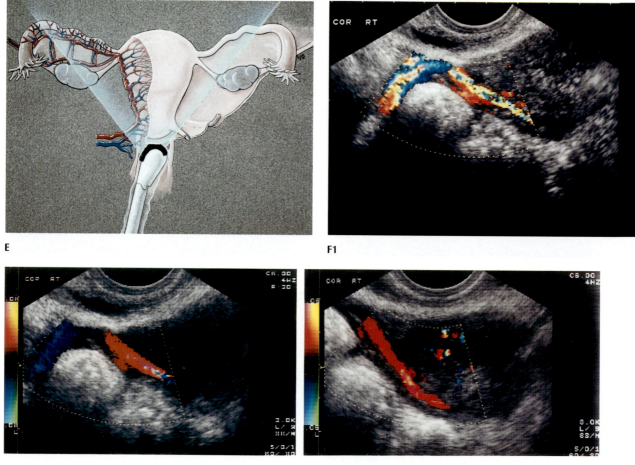

E

F1

F2

F3

FIGURE 3-4 *(continued)* **(E)** Diagram of transvaginal color Doppler sonographic (TV-CDS) depiction of uterine and adnexal vasculature. **(F)** TV-CDS shows the uterine artery and vein as they course into arcuate vessels. *(Figure continued.)*

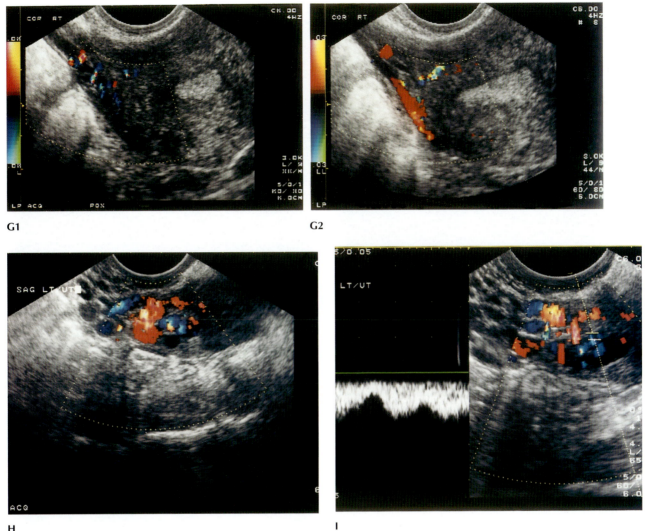

G1

G2

H

I

FIGURE 3-4 *(continued)* **(G)** Composite TV-CDS shows the main uterine vascularity and vessels within myometrium. **(H)** TV-CDS of distended uterine vessels. **(I)** Same as **H** showing venous flow within these parauterine vessels.

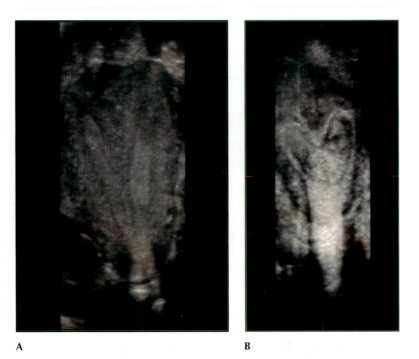

A   B

FIGURE 3-7 Three-dimensional sonography (3D US) of uterine malformation. **(A)** 3D US in mid-coronal plane showing two endometrial cavities and smooth configuration of uterine fundus, an indication of septated uterus. **(B)** Bicornuate uterus with hematometra within heart-shaped lumen.

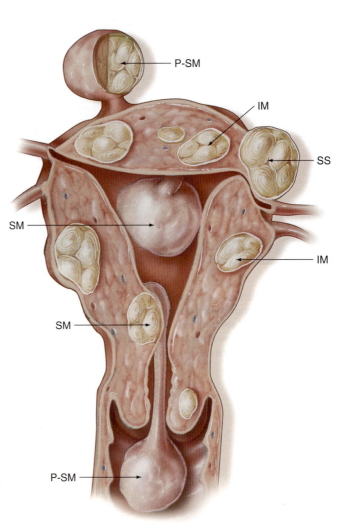

FIGURE 3-8 Different types of fibroids including P-SM, pedunculated submucosal fibroids; IM, intramural fibroids; SS, subserosal fibroids; and P-SS, pedunculated subserosal fibroids.

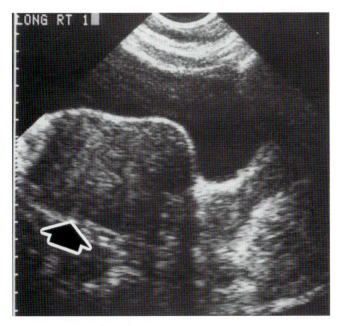

A

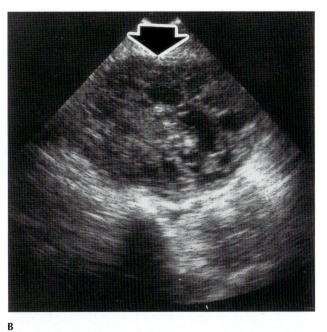

B

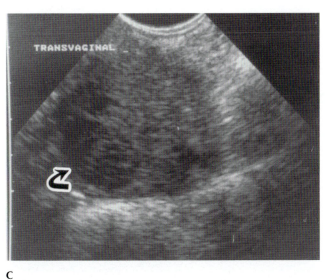

C

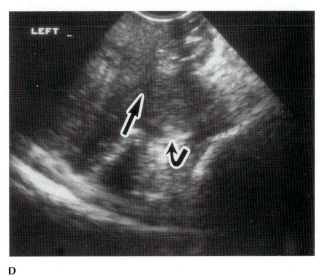

D

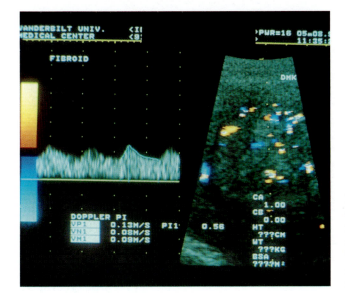

E

Figure 3-9 Fibroids. **(A)** TAS of large uterine fibroid (*arrow*) extending from uterine fundus. **(B)** Transverse TAS of degenerated fibroid (*arrow*) with cystic regions. **(C)** TVS of intramural fibroid appearing as hypoechoic area of the uterine corpus (*arrow*). **(D)** TVS of pedunculated subserosal fibroid (*curved arrow*) extending from the left uterine corpus by a broad pedicle (*straight arrow*). **(E)** TV-CDS of a vascular intramural fibroid. *(Figure continued.)*

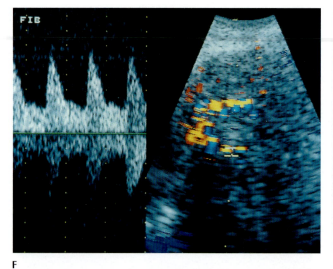

F

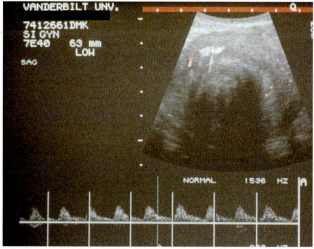

G

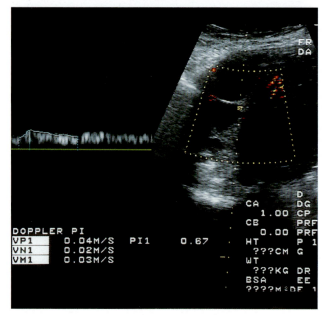

H

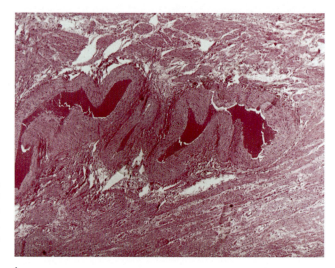

I

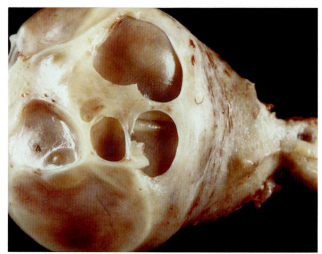

J

FIGURE 3-9 *(continued)* **(F)** TV-CDS of the vascular rim of a submucosal fibroid. **(G)** TV-CDS of a relatively hypovascular fibroid. **(H)** TVS of cystic mass within uterus containing low-velocity, low-impedance flow. **(I)** Gross specimen of mass shown in **H**. **(J)** Photomicrograph of specimen in **I** showing tortuous vessels with muscular media. This was found to be a leiomyosarcoma.

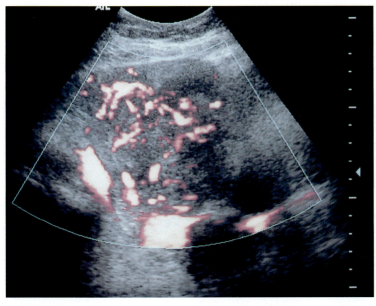

A

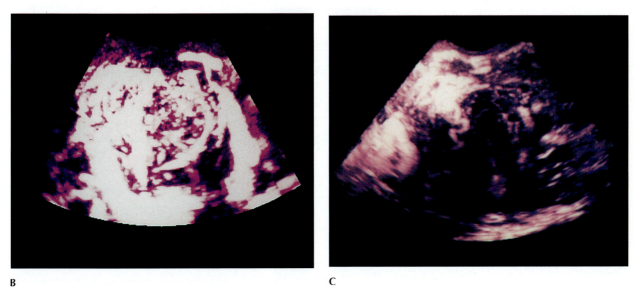

B   **C**

FIGURE 3-10 Three-dimensional color Doppler sonography (3D CDS) of fibroids pre- and postembolization. **(A)** Two-dimensional transabdominal color Doppler sonography (2D TA-CDS) of a large hypervascular fibroid prior to embolization. **(B)** 3D CDS of same patient in **A** showing hypervascularity. **(C)** 3D CDS one day after embolization showing markedly reduced flow.

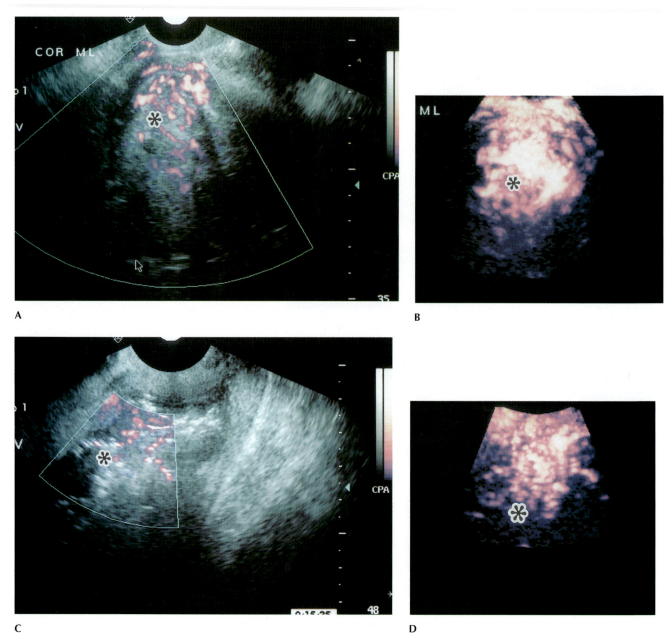

FIGURE 3-11 3D TV-CDS before and after fibroid embolization. **(A)** 2D TV-CDS of fibroid (*) in corpus showing rim of vascularity and central vascularity. **(B)** 3D TV-CDS showing the vascularity of the fibroid (*) before embolization. **(C)** 2D TV-CDS 1.5 days after embolization with Ivalon. There are echogenic foci representing the material used for embolization surrounding the fibroid (*). **(D)** 3D TV-CDS 1.5 days after embolization showing a marked reduction in fibroid flow (*).

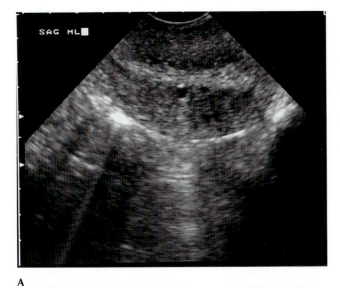

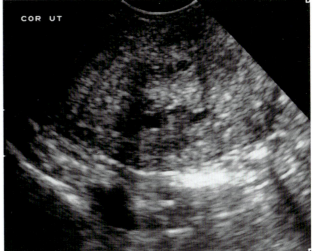

A

B

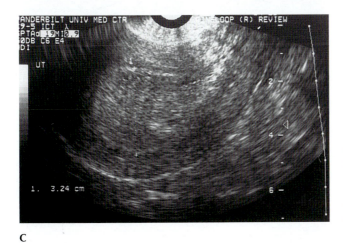

C

FIGURE 3-12 Disorders observed during tamoxifen therapy. **(A)** Long axis of normal endometrium with multiple cystic areas in the inner myometrium. These were thought to represent reactivated adenomyomas. **(B)** Short axis of normal endometrium showing cystic foci within the inner myometrium. **(C)** Markedly thickened endometrium in a patient on tamoxifen. Biopsy showed simple hyperplasia.

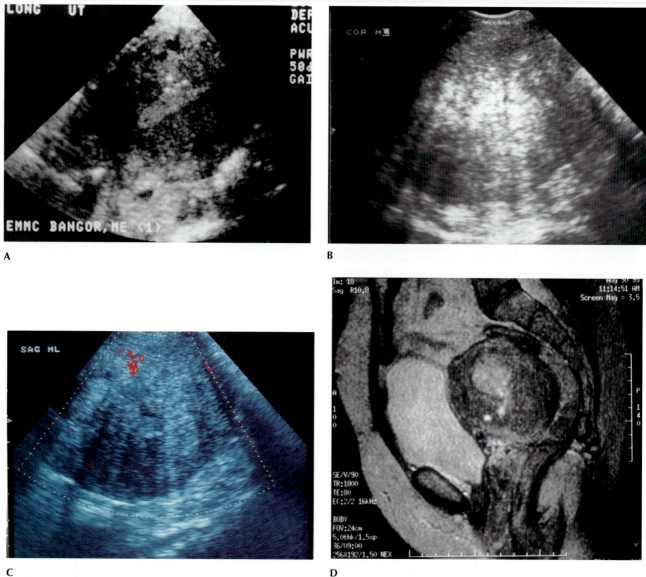

FIGURE 3-13 (A) Echogenic foci in the inner myometrium following dilation and curettage. (*Courtesy of Mary Warner, M.D.*) **(B)** TVS showing an irregular echogenic area in an enlarged, bulbous-appearing uterus. **(C)** TV-CDS of the same area as **B** showing scattered vessels within the echogenic myometrial area. **(D)** Magnetic resonance T2-weighted image shows foci of intense signal arising from intramyometrial hemorrhage within adenomyosis.

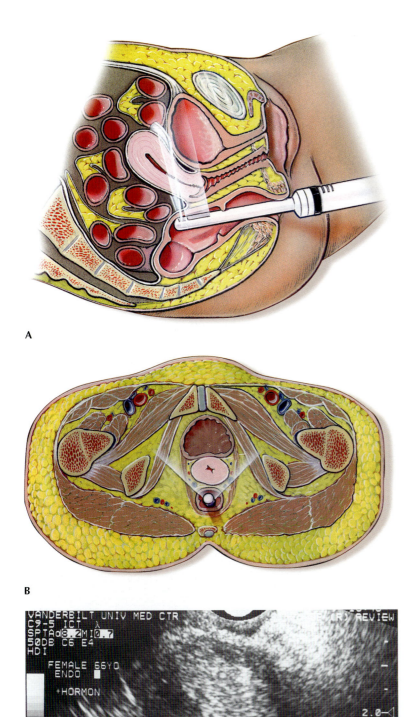

A

B

C

FIGURE 3-14 Transrectal sonographic (TRS) guidance. **(A)** Diagram showing field of transrectal biplane probe. The longitudinally oriented transducer array provides excellent delineation of the cervix in the long axis. **(B)** Diagram of TRS using axially oriented transducers at the tip of the probe provides confirmation of placement in both planes. Bladder distention assists in the sonographic demonstration of the cervix and corpus of the uterus by making the uterine plane more horizontal to the imaging plane. **(C)** TVS shows a focal area of increased echogenicity adjacent to the endometrium in a postmenopausal patient with bleeding. *(Figure continued.)*

53

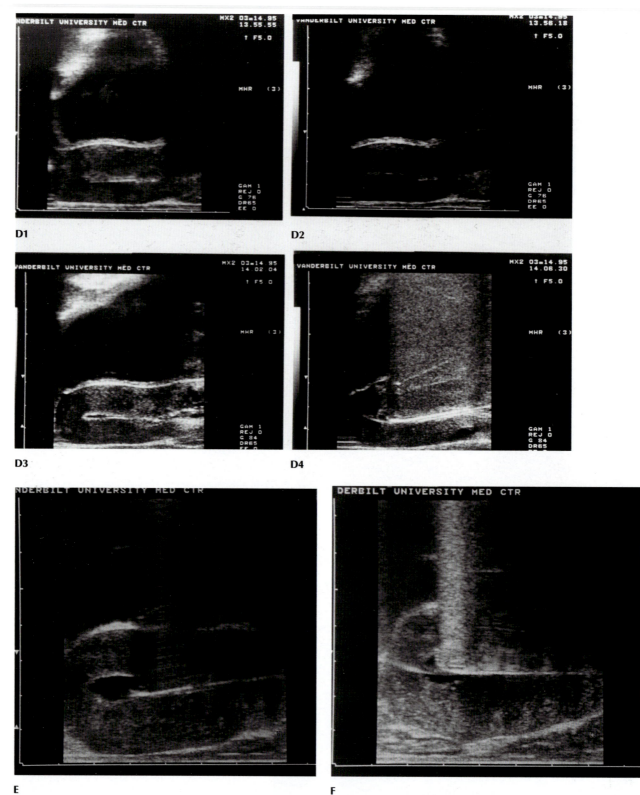

FIGURE 3-14 *(continued)* **(D)** Composite TRS showing passage of dilator into the uterine lumen. Curettage of the suspected area can be documented with TRS. **(E, F)** TRS shows location of curette during dilation and curettage of the posterior endometrium **(E)** and the anterior endometrium **(F)**. *(Figure continued.)*

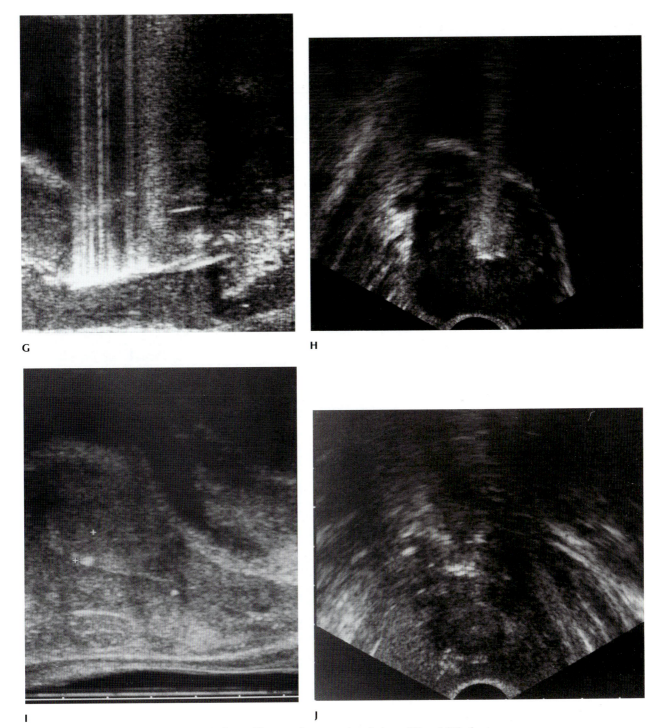

G

H

I

J

FIGURE 3-14 *(continued)* **(G, H)** TRS shows dilator at the external os in long **(G)** and **(H)** short axes. **(I, J)** TRS-guided circlage placement. The sutures are echogenic and appropriately placed within the upper cervix, as depicted on the long **(I)** and short **(J)** axes. The circular course of the circlage can be appreciated in the axial image. *(Figure continued.)*

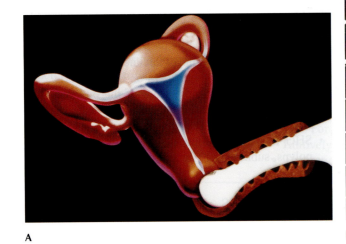

A

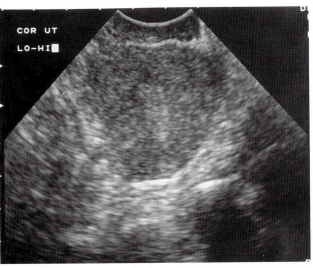

B

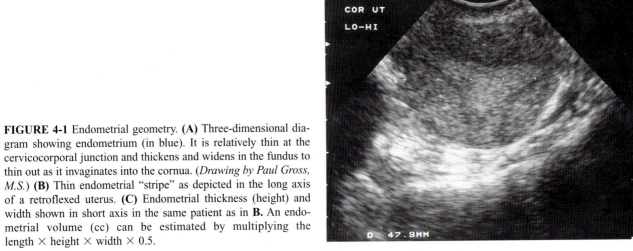

C

FIGURE 4-1 Endometrial geometry. **(A)** Three-dimensional diagram showing endometrium (in blue). It is relatively thin at the cervicocorporal junction and thickens and widens in the fundus to thin out as it invaginates into the cornua. (*Drawing by Paul Gross, M.S.*) **(B)** Thin endometrial "stripe" as depicted in the long axis of a retroflexed uterus. **(C)** Endometrial thickness (height) and width shown in short axis in the same patient as in **B.** An endometrial volume (cc) can be estimated by multiplying the length × height × width × 0.5.

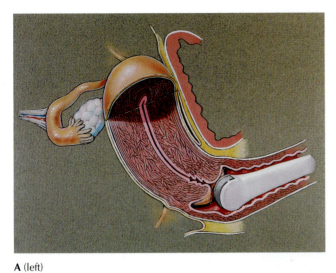

A (left)

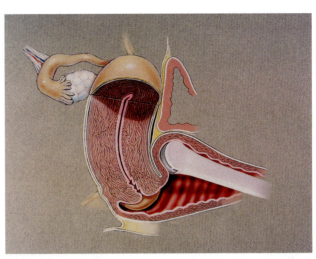

A (right)

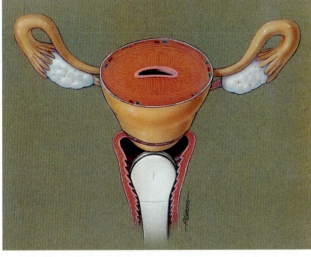

B

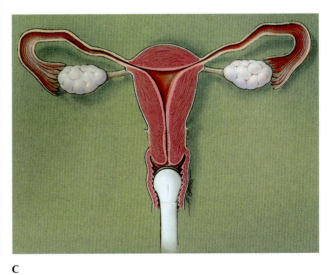

C

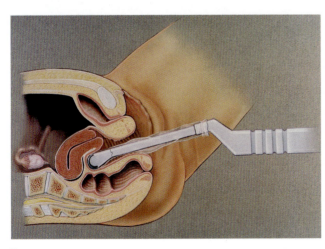

D

FIGURE 4-2 Transvaginal sonography (TVS) planes for depiction of the endometrium. (*Diagrams by Paul Gross, MS.*) **(A)** Long axis of an anteflexed uterus showing orientation of the endometrium to the transducer (*left*). The transducer can be advanced into the arterior fornix for better delineation of the endometrium (*right*). The opposite is true for retroflexed uteri. **(B)** Short-axis image of the endometrium. With pressure on the probe and placement of the probe head in the anterior fornix for an anteflexed uterus, the endometrium is imaged in its short axis. **(C)** Coronal view depicting "endometrial width." This plane is most readily obtained in a "neutral" positioned (neither ante- nor retroflexed) uterus. **(D)** Long axis of endometrium in a retroflexed uterus. With pressure on the posterior fornix, the endometrium becomes more horizontal to the transducer, allowing better detection.

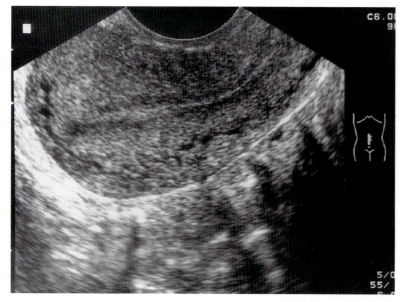

A

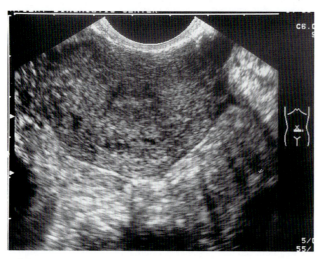

B (left)

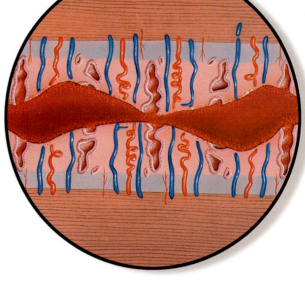

B (right)

FIGURE 4-3 Normal endometrium as depicted by TVS. **(A, B)** Long **(A)** and short **(B)** axes of early proliferative endometrium. TVS (**B,** *left*) and accompanying diagram show microscopic anatomy of the endometrium (**B,** *right*). (*Diagram by Paul Gross, MS.*) *(Figure continued.)*

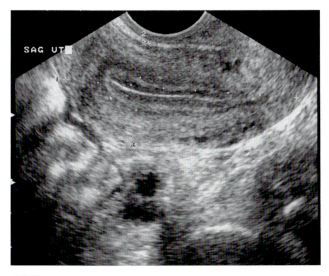

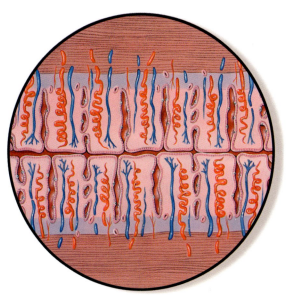

C (left)

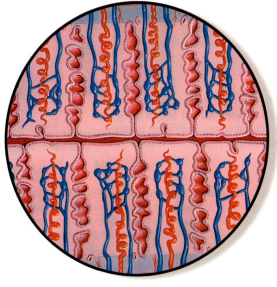

C (right)

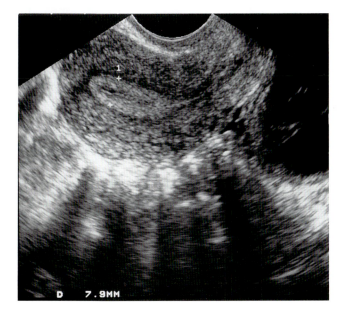

D (left)

D (right)

FIGURE 4-3 *(continued)* **(C)** Long axis of the endometrium in midcycle *(left)*. A multilayered appearance is seen with the outer echogenic interface representing basalis, the inner layer functionalis, and the median echo from refluxed mucus. Diagram of corresponding microscopic anatomy *(right)*. The glandular elements and stroma enlarge, whereas the basal layer (light blue) remains constant. **(D)** Luteal phase endometrium appearing as thick (8 mm), regular, and echogenic *(left)*. Diagram showing thickened stroma and distended glands *(right)*. *(Figure continued.)*

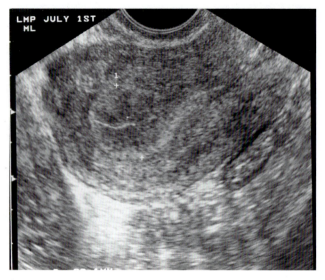

A

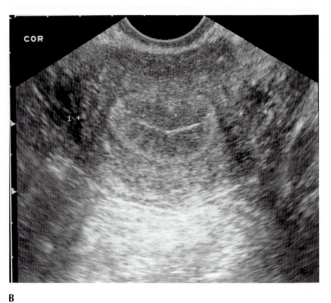

B

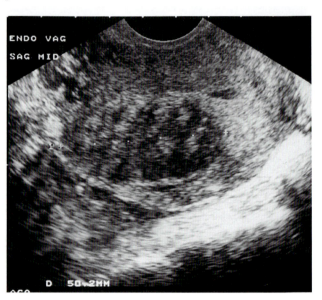

C

FIGURE 4-4 Dysfunctional bleeding. **(A)** Thick endometrium in a premenopausal woman presenting with bleeding. The endometrium (*between cursors*) measures 22 mm. **(B)** Same as in **A** on short axis. Biopsy was negative for hyperplasia. **(C)** Submucosal fibroid displacing endometrium in a patient with dysfunctional uterine bleeding.

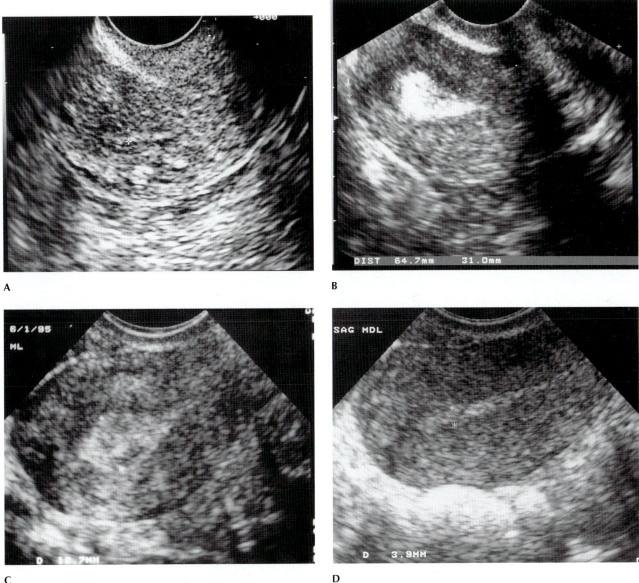

FIGURE 4-5 Disorders observed with hormone replacement therapy (HRT) and selective estrogen receptor modulators. **(A)** Thin endometrium (between cursors) in a patient on HRT due to endometrial atrophy. **(B)** Thick and echogenic endometrium in a patient on HRT due to endometrial hyperplasia. The echogenic material represented abundant mucus surrounding a small polyp. **(C)** Thick and irregular endometrium in a patient with bleeding on HRT. Hyperplasia was found on biopsy. **(D)** Follow-up TVS of patient shown in **C** after 4 months. After dilation and curretage, the endometrium is thin and regular.

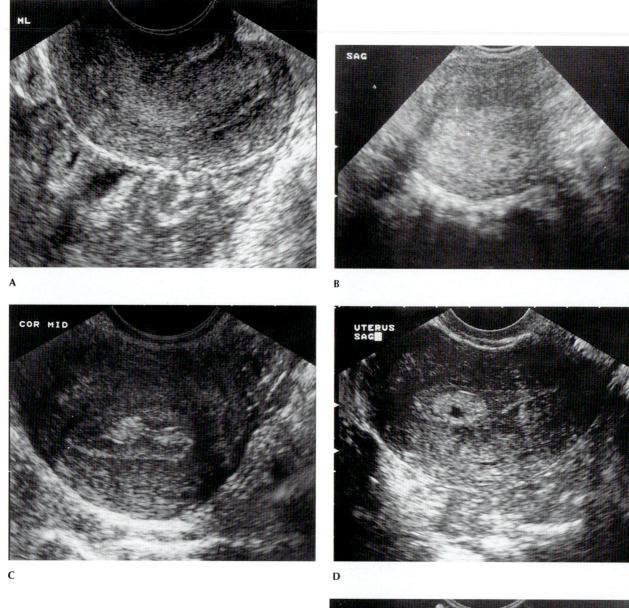

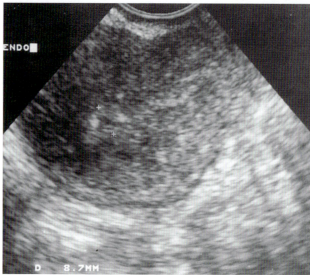

FIGURE 4-6 TVS findings in postmenopausal bleeding. **(A)** Atrophic endometrium in a postmenopausal woman with a retroflexed uterus. **(B)** Hyperplastic endometrium (*between cursors*) in a woman on tamoxifen. Myometrial cysts are also present. **(C)** Echogenic polyp insinuated between relatively hypoechoic endometrial layers. **(D)** An echogenic polyp contains a cystic area, representing distended glands within the polyp. **(E)** Thick and irregular endometrium (*between cursors*). Hyperplasia was found at biopsy.

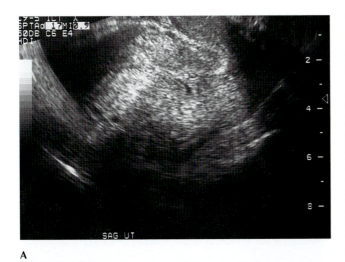

A

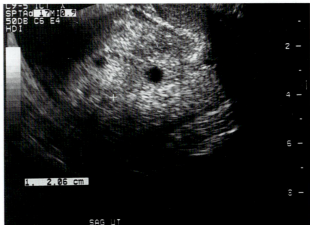

B

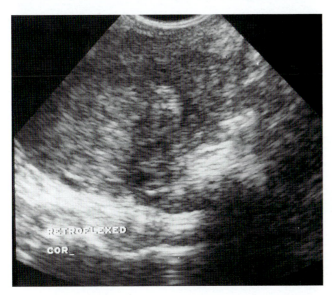

C

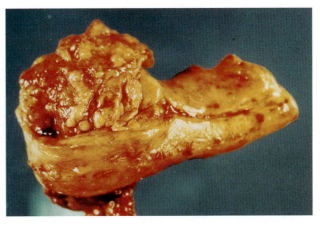

D

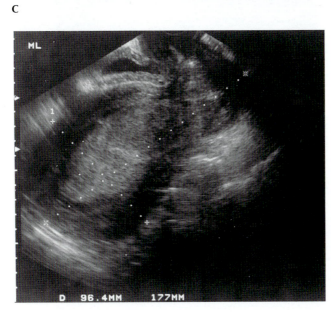

E

FIGURE 4-7 Endometrial cancer. **(A, B)** Long-axis images of a polypoid mass surrounded by a thin sliver of intraluminal fluid. This tumor occupied the entire uterine lumen and was found to be an endometroid cancer. **(C, D)** Invasive endometrial cancer extending to uterine serosa in the fundal region. **(D)** Picture of gross specimen showing tumor extending to serosa. **(E)** Noninvasive endometrial cancer appearing as bulky tumor that markedly distends the uterine lumen. Because the inner hypoechoic myometrium was seen to be intact on TVS, this was correctly determined to be noninvasive. *(Figure continued.)*

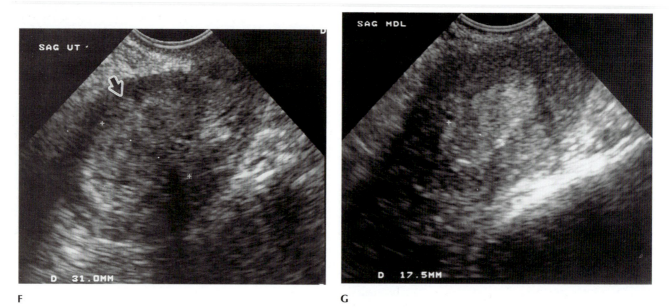

F

G

FIGURE 4-7 *(continued)* **(F)** Invasive endometrial cancer. Compared to the patient shown in **E,** there is disruption of the junctional zone *(arrow)* in the invasive tumor. **(G)** Focally invasive endometrial cancer in a patient on hormone replacement therapy. There is a "tongue" of echogenic tissue disrupting the inner myometrium, indicating that this is locally invasive.

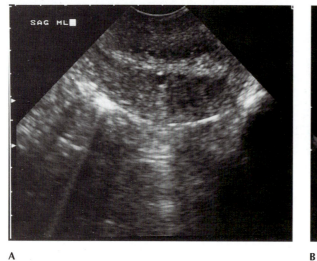

A

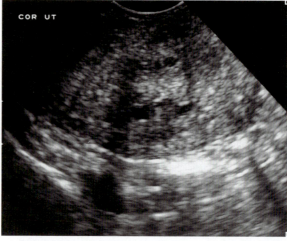

B

FIGURE 4-8 Disorders observed during tamoxifen therapy. **(A)** Long axis of normal endometrium with multiple cystic areas in the inner myometrium. These are thought to represent reactivated adenomyomas. **(B)** Short axis of normal endometrium showing cystic foci within the inner myometrium. **(C)** Markedly thickened endometrium in a patient on tamoxifen. Biopsy showed simple hyperplasia.

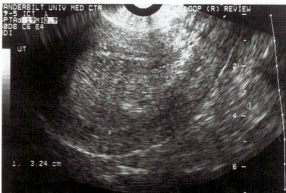

C

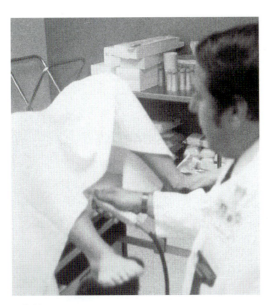

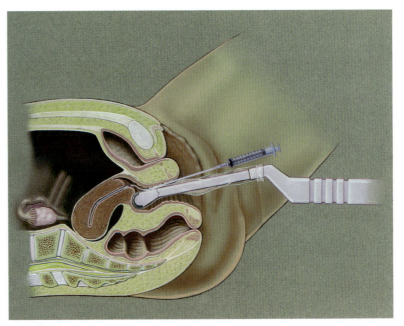

A (left)   **A** (right)

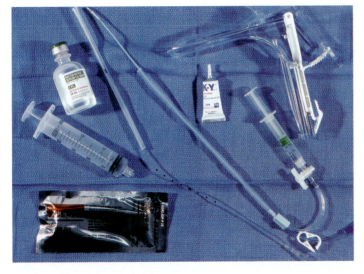

B

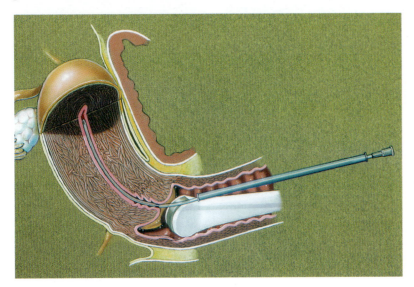

FIGURE 4-9 Sonohysterography (SHG): instrumentation and technique. (**A,** *left*) Patient on pelvic exam table ready for SHG. The patient's legs are supported in the stirrups. The examiner sits on a moveable stool during insertion and then stands to see the monitor during injection. (**A,** *right*) Catheter and transducer in place for SHG. (**B**) "Set-up" tray for SHG includes speculum, catheters, saline, cleaning solution, and swabs. An open-lipped speculum is preferred to allow for grasping the catheter and removing the speculum once the catheter is in place. An H/S catheter and a Tampa catheter are shown. (**C**) Tampa catheter as a flexible catheter and an introducer. Before its insertion, the catheter is flushed with saline. The catheter is then withdrawn into the introducer. When the introducer is placed on the external os, the catheter is advanced through the introducer. *(Figure continued.)*

C

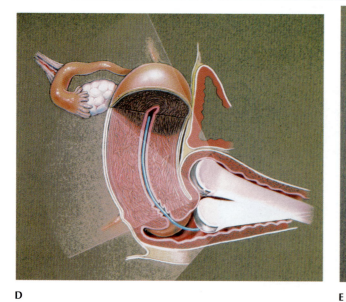

D

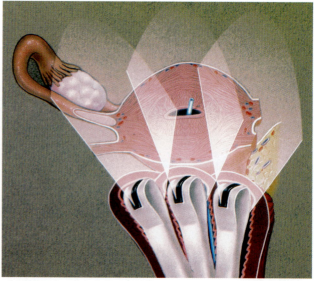

E

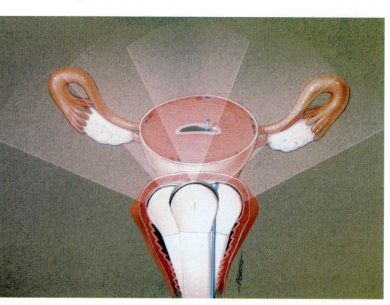

FIGURE 4-9 *(continued)* **(D, E, F)** Scanning maneuvers used for SHG. In the sagittal plane **(D)**, the transducer/probe is directed anteriorly for an anteflexed uterus and posteriorly for a retroflexed uterus. The transducer probe is moved from side to side for delineation of the endometrium in the semi-sagittal **(E)** and semi-axial **(F)** planes. *(Figure continued.)*

F

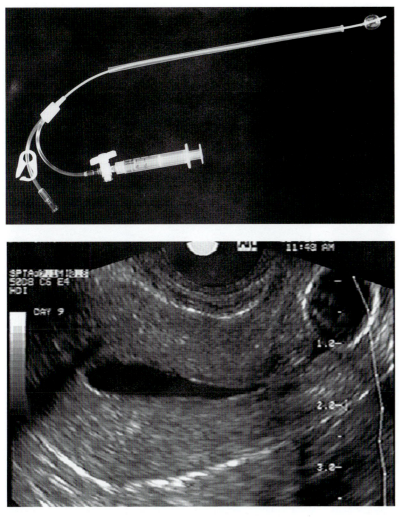

G

FIGURE 4-9 *(continued)* **(G)** H/S catheter with distended balloon *(top)*. SHG with H/S catheter *(bottom)*. The distended balloon is within the endocervical canal. *(Figure continued.)*

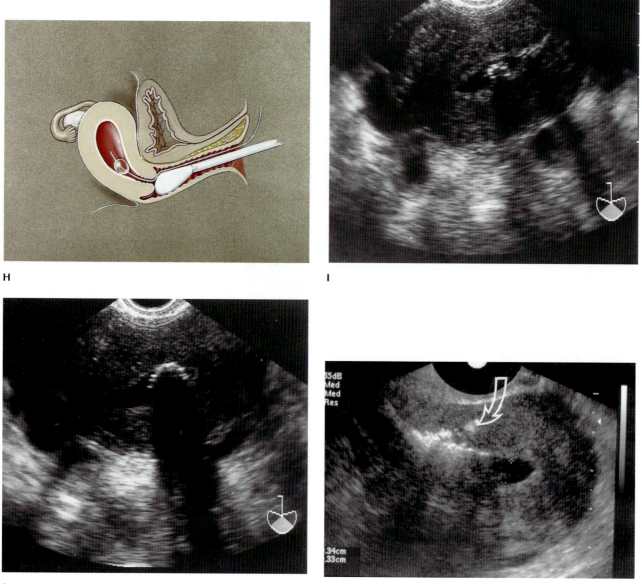

H

I

J

K

FIGURE 4-9 *(continued)* **(H)** SHG using pediatric Foley catheter. Any balloon can cause artifacts when placed in the uterine cavity. Balloons are best filled with water and kept at or below the internal os. **(I)** SHG using balloon catheter. This image was taken during initial instillation. **(J)** Same as in **I** but later and with more distention. Note that the air-containing balloon blocks delineation of the distal endometrial interface. **(K)** Asherman's syndrome. A retroverted sagittal uterus with supracervical synechiae in an amenorrheic woman with occult menses through patent tubes and cyclic pain. There is a small amount of air trapped above the synechiae, producing gas attenuation across half the cavity. A straight catheter penetrated the synechiae, but infusion of saline rapidly created bright myometrial echoes *(arrow)* due to saline being forced into tiny sinuses (myometrial psuedo diverticulae) at the point of cavitary obstruction. The fundal cavity is normal, with proliferative endometrium. *(Figure continued.)*

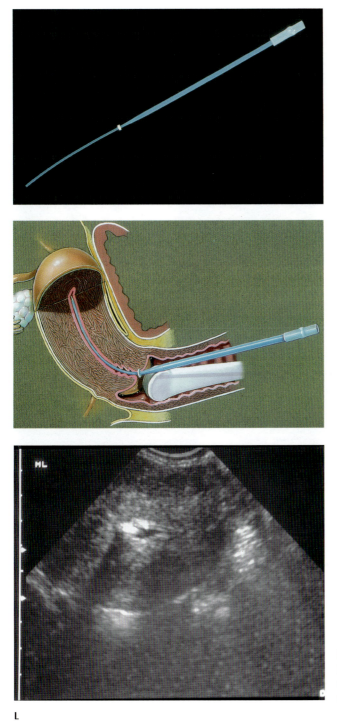

FIGURE 4-9 *(continued)* **(L)** Soules insemination catheter (*top*) is less flexible than the Tampa catheter and can be used to cannulate tougher cervices. SHG using the Soules catheter (*center and bottom*). The echogenic interface is the catheter. *(Figure continued.)*

L

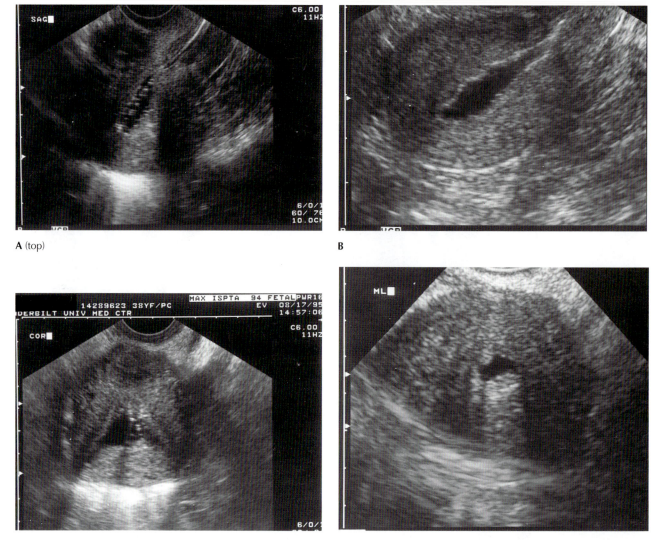

A (top)

B

A (bottom)

C

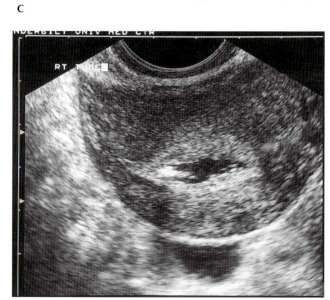

FIGURE 4-11 (A) Long- (*top*) and short- (*bottom*) axis images from SHG during the follicular phase. Note the thin and regular endometrium. The bubbles within the lumen are due to mucus. **(B, C)** Long-axis **(B)** and short-axis **(C)** images taken during SHG in the early secretory phase. Note the mild serration of the inner endometrium as seen on the short axis. This has been termed an endometrial "wrinkle." **(D)** Short-axis image from SHG during mid-secretory phase, showing mild thickening and irregularity typically seen in midluteal phase endometrium. *(Figure continued.)*

D

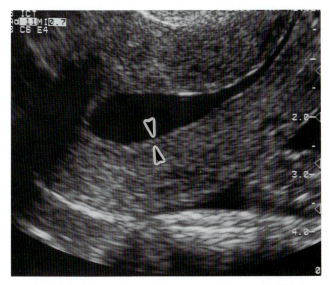

E

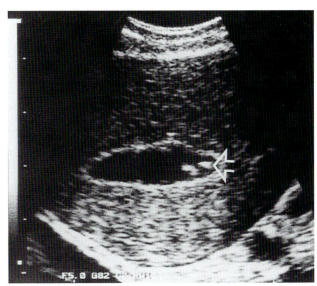

F

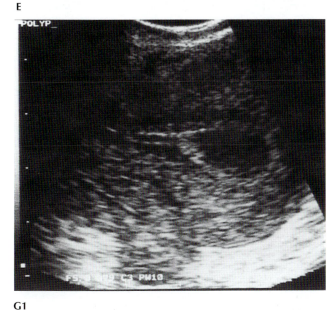

G1

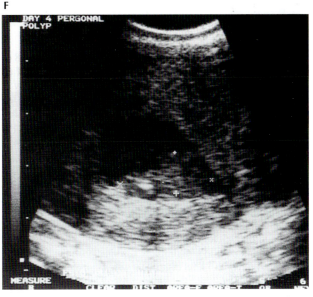

G2

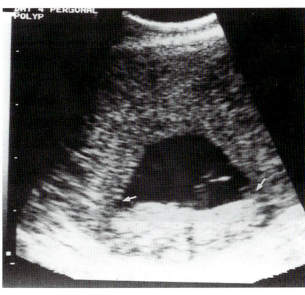

G3

FIGURE 4-11 *(continued)* **(E)** Normal proliferative endometrium, day 6 (4 days after completion of menses, during saline infusion). The very smooth surface provides a sharply etched interface between the layers during the proliferative phase, making this an excellent time to demonstrate intracavitary abnormalities. *Arrowheads* point to the minimally expanded functionalis layer. **(F)** Proliferative endometrium, day 10. A transverse view of tiny tufts of proliferative endometrium (*arrow*) in the left cornu of a 35-year-old woman with habitual abortion due to inadequate luteal progesterone effect, the later correction of which resulted in term pregnancy. The rest of the endometrium is normal with a typically smooth surface. These may represent focally persistent functionalis due to inadequate progesterone effect. **(G)** Midproliferative endometrium, day 4 of Pergonal (Serono Laboratories, Randolph, MA) (estradiol = 120 pg/mL). This illustrates a normal to midproliferative phase endometrium containing an apparent fundal mass despite a normal biopsy in the previous cycle. Note that the typical layered effect of advancing proliferation is best seen in the unseparated layers. Endometrial fluid defines endometrial thickness and contour, but it can obscure such subtle hormone effects. **(G1)** Apparently sequestered due to the sharp retroversion of the uterus, the "polyp" consists of residual menstrual effluvium, which is washed out. **(G2)** During sonohysterography, shown in the dependent transverse fundus (cornu inferior). Endometrial polyps are virtually never entirely hypoechoic. **(G3)** The normal transverse fundus after instillation of saline and expulsion of debris. Arrows indicate the tubal ostia. Identification of the ostia is important to confirm a normal cavitary shape. There is scant floating debris in the left cornu. The gain has been turned up to demonstrate the clarity of the fluid. *(Figure continued.)*

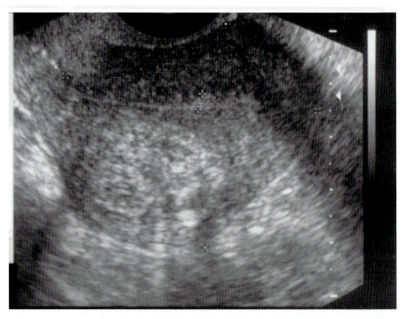

Q (top)

FIGURE 4-11 *(continued)* **(Q)** Postmenstrual endometrium in a retroverted uterus with an anterior myoma (*top*) that approaches the cavity: is it submucosal or intramural? This 45-year-old woman has midcycle bleeding and an appropriate 3-mm endometrial thickness after menses. The cavity is normal and the myoma is clearly intramural (*bottom*), suggesting that the midcycle bleeding is from ovarian dysfunction. The bubble present in Fig. 4-9N has now escaped, revealing the internal os. *(Figure continued.)*

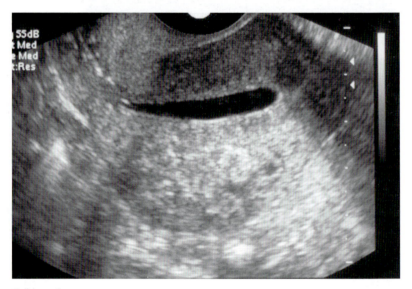

Q (bottom)

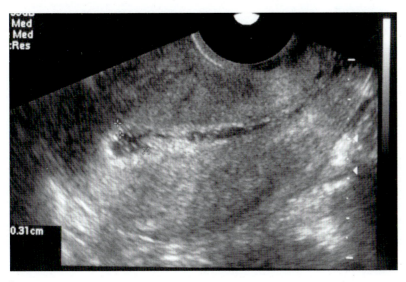

R

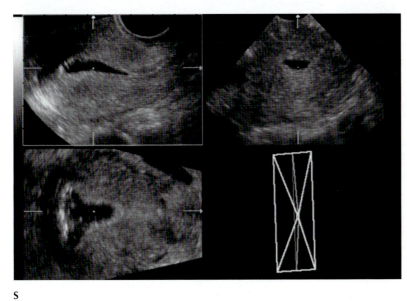

S

FIGURE 4-11 *(continued)* **(R)** A 49-year-old woman with menometrorrhagia and no evidence of recent ovulation in the ovaries. The unenhanced endometrium is 7.5 mm thick and the anteverted uterus is otherwise normal and nontender. Saline infusion of the uterus demonstrates an irregular surface and focal immovable thickening on the posterior mid wall. **(S)** After treatment with 14 days of progestin and a 3-day withdrawal bleed, the unenhanced endometrium in the same uterus as in **R** is now 4 mm, and a 3D saline infusion demonstrated uniform thickness in the *(clockwise from upper left)* sagittal, transverse, and coronal orthogonal planes. The white dot in midcavity correlates with the same point in all three images. Because the abnormality was shed after progestin, a biopsy was not performed, and cycle control was prompt with low-dose oral contraceptives.

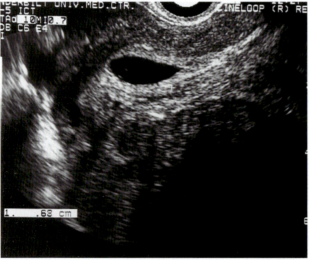

A

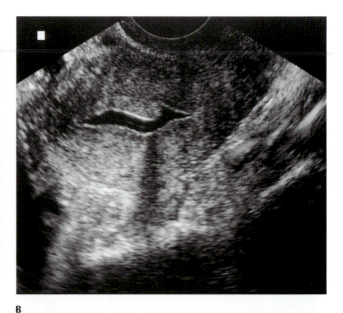

B

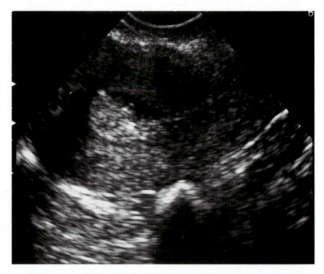

C

 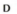

D

FIGURE 4-12 Hyperplasia. **(A)** TVS showing minimal thickening of the anterior endometrium (*arrowhead*). **(B)** SHG of patient in **A** confirming asymmetric thickening of the anterior layer of endometrium. Biopsy showed proliferative changes. **(C)** Perimenopausal patient with a clinical history of menometrorrhagia. Saline infusion SHG depicts a thickened homogenous endometrium surrounding the sonolucent fluid instillation. The endometrium measures 6.8 and 4.9 mm, respectively. Pathology from the endometrial biopsy revealed simple hyperplasia without atypia. The bleeding history and the lack of an identifiable corpus luteum are the only means of distinguishing hyperplastic from secretory endometrium, except for biopsy. Compare with **B**. **(D)** Focal endometrial thickening. This image demonstrates the importance of SHG; if only the posterior wall endometrium had been biopsied, a false-negative result would have occurred. The focally thick endometrium was biopsied, which revealed disordered proliferative changes. **(E)** Endometrial hyperplasia. Sagittal uterus in an obese 41-year-old woman with anovulatory bleeding showing focal simple hyperplasia on the posterior wall, marked "1." Biopsy of the anterior wall revealed "normal" proliferation. *(Figure continued.)*

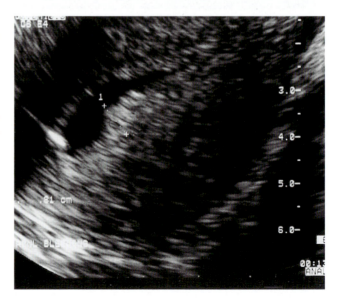

E

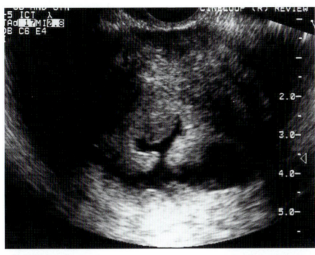

F1

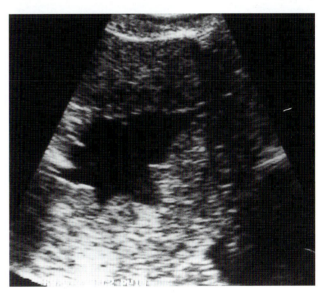

F2

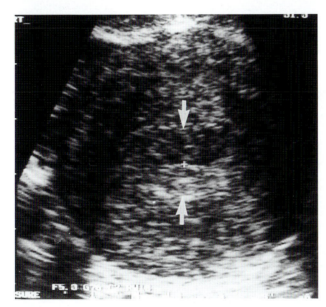

G1

G2

FIGURE 4-12 *(continued)* **(F)** Endometrial hyperplasia. **(F1)** Fundal polypoid complex hyperplasia, diagnosed by office biopsy, in a 46-year-old woman with anemia due to prolonged anovulatory uterine bleeding. In the transverse view, the posterior wall (inferior) is also irregular, but it is not clearly seen in this view. **(F2)** Sagittal view of the same patient 4 months later, after treatment with cyclic medroxyprogesterone acetate (MPA) to allow organized monthly withdrawal (day 4 of the progestin). Note the typically jagged endometrium in this artificial secretory phase, confirmed by biopsy. The hyperplasia has completely regressed, and her cycle is controlled with monthly progestin. **(G)** Endometrial hyperplasia. The acute effect of high-dose progestin on hyperplasia is to halt proliferation and stop bleeding. **(G1)** This is an example of decidualized endometrial hyperplasia (16 mm between *arrows*) after 6 days of 80 mg of megestrol acetate per day. **(G2)** A sagittal view of the same uterus with infusion demonstrates the typical jagged effect of progestin superimposed on anovulatory proliferation or hyperplasia. After 1 month of continuous progestin, the bilayer endometrium regressed to 5 mm with no bleeding and no curettage was required. Cyclic progestins thereafter prevented further hyperplasia. *(Figure continued.)*

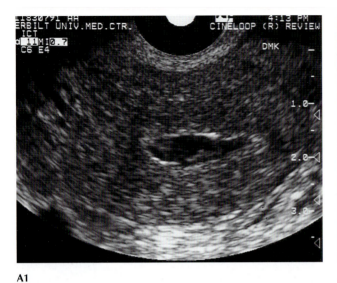

A1

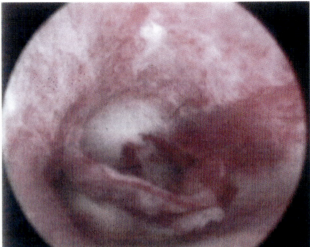

A2

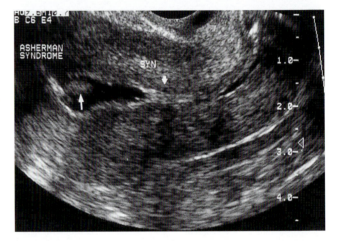

B

FIGURE 4-14 (A) SHG and hysteroscopy showing adhesions. **(A1)** SHG showing adhesions within the endometrial lumen. **(A2)** Hysteroscopy of intraluminal adhesions. (*Hysteroscopic image courtesy of E. Eisenberg, M.D.*) **(B)** Synechiae. A 37-year-old woman who had had an elective abortion presented with infertility. At midcycle the endometrium was thin and irregular. Infusion reveals partial agglutination (SYN) of the lower segment that admits saline and a right corneal polyp (*longer arrow*). The walls were easily separated by blunt hysteroscopic lysis of adhesions in this case. Polypectomy was also performed. She conceived 6 months later. (*Figure continued.*)

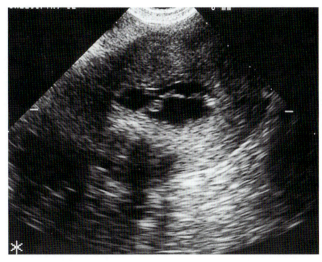

C1

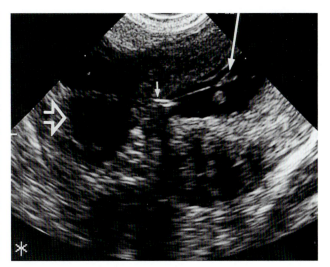

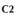

C2

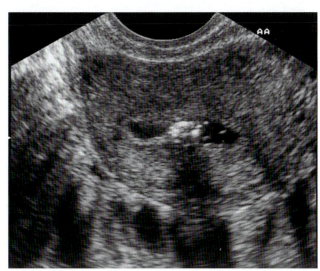

D1

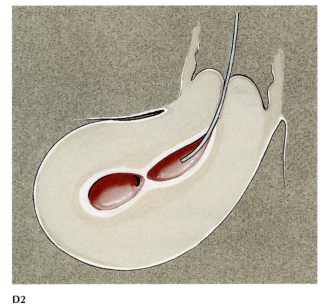

D2

FIGURE 4-14 *(continued)* **(C)** Synechiae. **(C1)** A mesh of synechiae crosses the upper cavity of the 32-year-old nulliparous woman who underwent dilation and curettage (D&C) during surgery for an ectopic pregnancy. She has normal, regular menses but has had 5 years of infertility with one patent normal tube. It is day 17 of the cycle, and the endometrium is somewhat poorly defined, despite being postovulatory. **(C2)** The synechiae *(long arrow)* can be seen to extend into the recess of the right (damaged) tube (at the *short arrow*). The saline often makes a bright artifact at the tubal orifice *(short arrow)*. On the reader's left the right ovary *(open arrow)* contains two corpora lutea. **(D)** SHG and diagram of adhesions. **(D1)** SHG with typical "bow tie" configuration of an adhesion. **(D2)** Diagram of an endometrial adhesion.

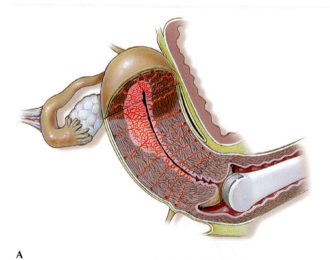

A

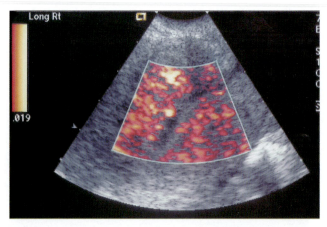

B

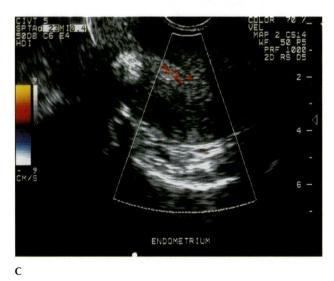

C

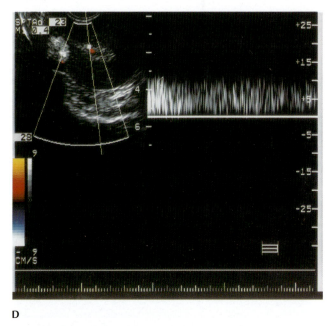

D

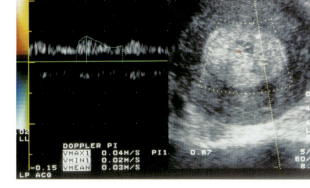

E

FIGURE 4-15 Transvaginal color Doppler sonography (TV-CDS) of endometrial disorders. **(A)** Diagram showing increased vascularity in an endometrial tumor. (*Drawing by Paul Gross, M.S.*) **(B)** Normal TV-CDS showing spiral arterioles within the basal layer of the endometrium. **(C, D)** Increased flow in women presenting with bleeding. The TV-CDS shows venous-like flow arising from within the endometrium. (*Courtesy of C. Peery, M.D.*) **(E)** Polyp containing several vessels with low impedance. (*Figure continued.*)

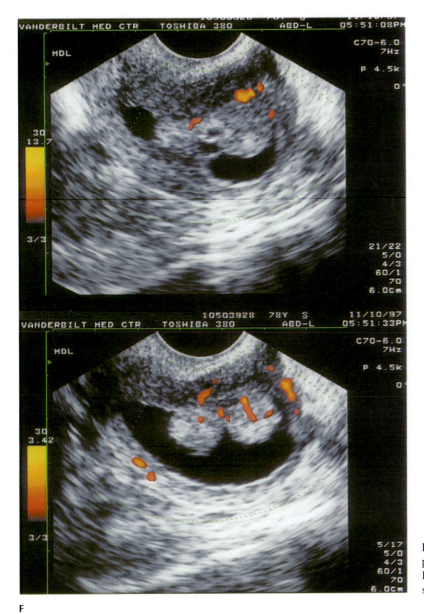

F

FIGURE 4-15 *(continued)* **(F)** Two views of polypoid endometrial cancer with feeding vessels. Intraluminal fluid was present due to cervical stenosis. *(Figure continued.)*

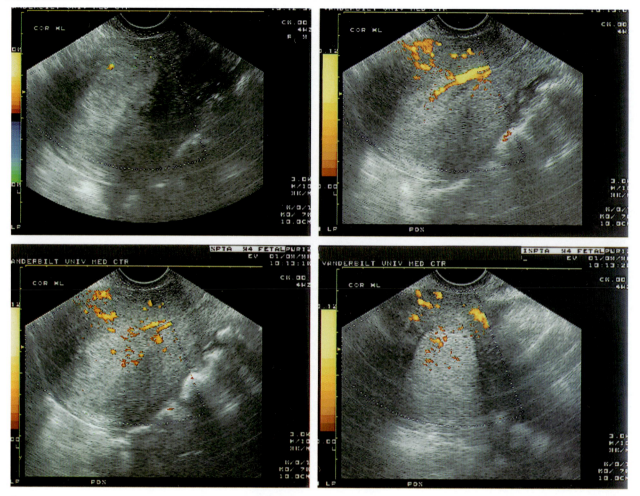

G

FIGURE 4-15 *(continued)* **(G)** Composite TV-CDS of a woman on tamoxifen presenting with bleeding. There is marked thickening of the endometrium and hypervascularity. Simple hyperplasia was found at biopsy.

5 PELVIC MASSES

OVERVIEW

- Transabdominal sonography (TAS) provides an overview; transvaginal sonography (TVS) depicts details.
- For some large pelvic or pelvoabdominal masses, such as fibroids, TAS is best.
- The important features of a pelvic mass include:
  - Organ of origin: uterine, ovarian, tubal, bowel
  - Internal contents: i.e., completely cystic, mostly cystic with solid areas, papillary excrescence, solid with echogenic components
  - Associated findings, such as ascites, pelvocalycectasis
- It is vital to incorporate patient's age, presenting symptoms, and pelvic exam findings with the sonographic features to derive most likely diagnoses.
- Physiologic masses such as hemorrhagic corpora lutea are common in women of childbearing age. Therefore, it is important to perform serial studies (repeat in 4–6 weeks) to assess for regression. A significant percentage (50%–70%) of pelvic masses that do not regress are neoplasms.
- TVS can be used for guided aspiration of some pelvic masses, such as those created by ovarian remnants.
- TVS-guided aspiration of certain pelvic masses, such as physiologic cysts thought to be the cause of pelvic pain or tubo-ovarian abscesses containing pus, can be curative.

DIFFERENTIAL DIAGNOSIS

- *See Figures 5-1 and 5-2.*
- As mentioned previously, sonographic evaluation of a pelvic mass includes assessment of its organ of origin, internal consistency, associated findings, and, in some cases, flow/vascularity assessment.
- The differential diagnosis can usually be narrowed down to one or two entities based on a combination of clinical and sonographic findings (Tables 5-1 and 5-2).

OVARIAN MASSES

- *See Figures 5-3 through 5-7.*
- Most common are physiologic masses arising from hemorrhage within a corpus luteum or continued fluid collection within a hydropic follicle.
- Age is an important factor in determining diagnostic possibilities. A large cystic mass in a postmenopausal woman is most likely a cystadenoma, while pelvic masses in younger women tend to be physiologic.
- Dermoid cysts have a variable sonographic appearance.
  - Some contain echogenic sebum and/or calcifications.
  - 15% are bilateral.
  - Some dermoid cysts are small, intraovarian, and appear as echogenic masses within the ovary.

TABLE 5-1 Sonographic Differential Diagnoses of Pelvic Masses*

CYSTIC	COMPLEX	SOLID
Completely cystic	**Predominantly cystic**	**Uterine**
Physiologic ovarian cysts	Cystadenomas	Leiomyoma (sarcoma)
Cystadenomas	Tubo-ovarian abscess	Endometrial carcinoma, sarcoma
Hydrosalpinx	Ectopic pregnancy	
Endometrioma	Cystic teratoma	**Extrauterine**
Paraovarian cyst		Solid ovarian tumor
Hydatid cyst of Morgagni	**Predominantly solid**	
	Cystadenoma (carcinoma)	
Multiple	Germ cell tumor	
Endometriomas		
Multiple follicular cysts		
Septated		
Cystadenoma (carcinoma)		
Mucinous		
Serous		
Papillary		

*Based on most common appearance.

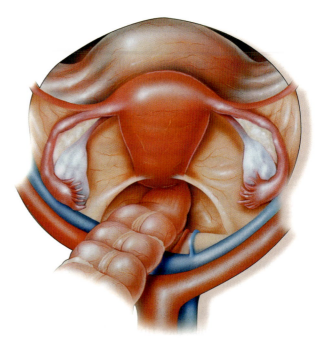

FIGURE 5-1 Pelvic organs as seen by pelvic surgeon from above. The bladder is shown at the top, with the uterus between the sigmoid colon and bladder. The broad ligament surrounds the ovaries and tube. The round ligament and proximal tube are adjacent to each other in the fundal regions of the uterus.

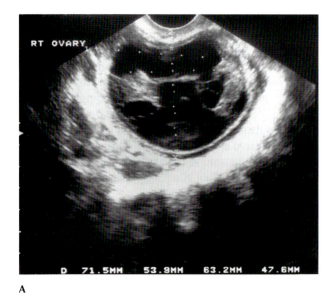

A

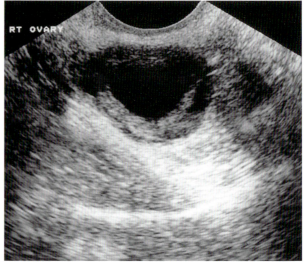

B

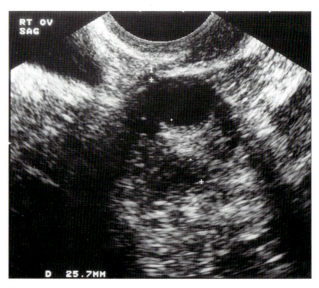

C

FIGURE 5-2 Spontaneous regression of complex cystic mass. **(A)** Transvaginal sonogram (TVS) showing a cystic mass within the right ovary containing irregular solid areas and septations. **(B)** Follow-up TVS 2 months later showing regression. Only a focal area of thickening remains. **(C)** Follow-up 1 year later showing residual cyst.

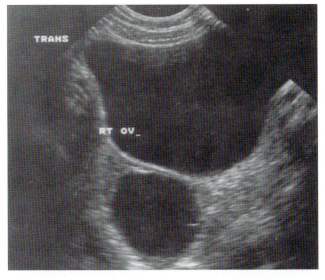

A

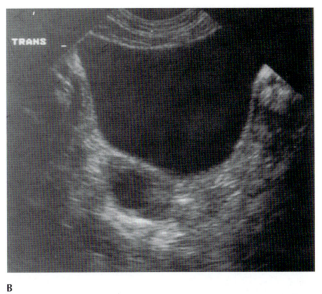

B

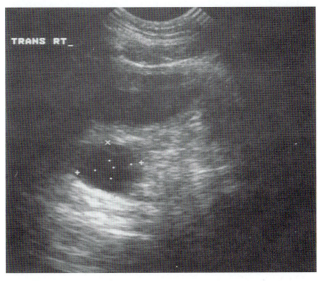

C

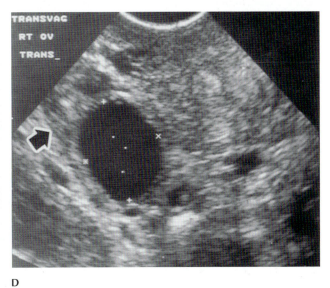

D

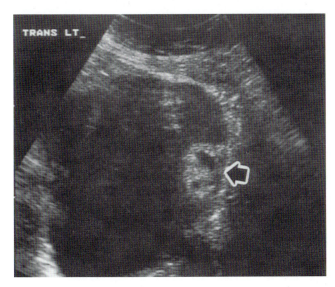

E

FIGURE 5-3 Completely cystic masses. **(A)** Longitudinal transabdominal sonogram (TAS) of completely cystic mass. **(B)** Same patient as in **A**, 1 month later, demonstrating complete resolution. **(C)** TAS of cystic right-adnexal mass (*between cursors*). **(D)** TVS of **C** showing follicular cyst (*between cursors*) within right ovary with a thin wall. Surrounding ovarian tissue (*arrow*) is compressed by cyst. **(E)** Transverse sonogram demonstrating predominantly cystic mass surrounding left ovary (*arrow*), representing a peritoneal cyst. *(Figure continued.)*

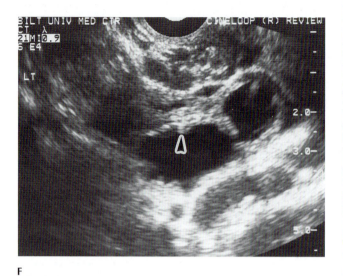

F

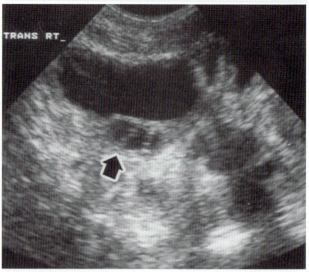

G

FIGURE 5-3 *(continued)* **(F)** TVS of cystic mass with a small intra-luminal projection *(arrow)* that represents an endosalpingeal fold within a hydrosalpinx. **(G)** TVS of luteal cyst demonstrating a wall thicker than that of a follicular cyst and a rim of ovarian tissue containing several immature follicles *(arrow)* surrounding cyst. **(H)** TVS of ruptured hemorrhagic corpus luteum cyst *(large arrow)* surrounded by echogenic clotted blood in cul-de-sac *(curved arrow).* *(Figure continued.)*

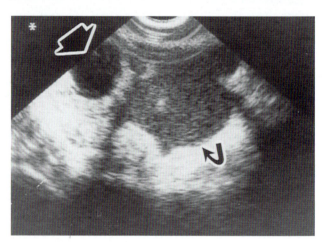

H

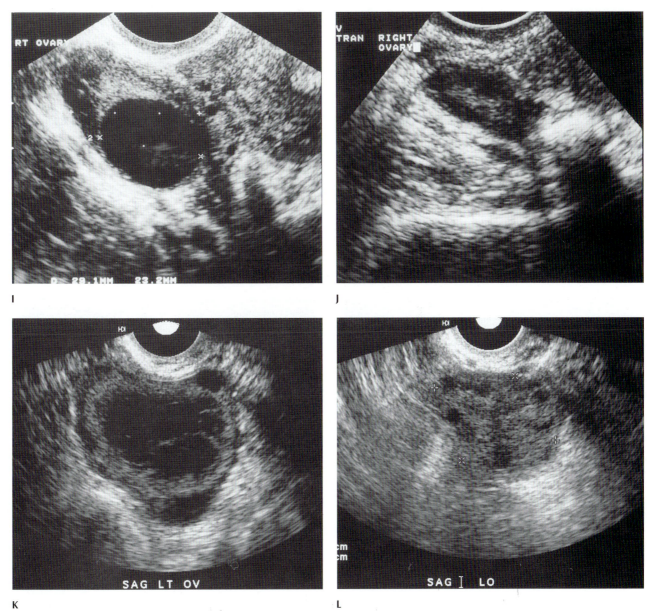

FIGURE 5-3 *(continued)* **(I)** TVS of smooth-walled ovarian cyst. **(J)** Same patient as in **I** after 5 weeks. There has been complete regression of the physiologic cyst. **(K)** Hemorrhagic corpus luteum within the left ovary containing fibrin strands appearing as a web-like complex of thin, branching linear interfaces. **(L)** Same patient as in **K**, 6 weeks later, showing complete regression.

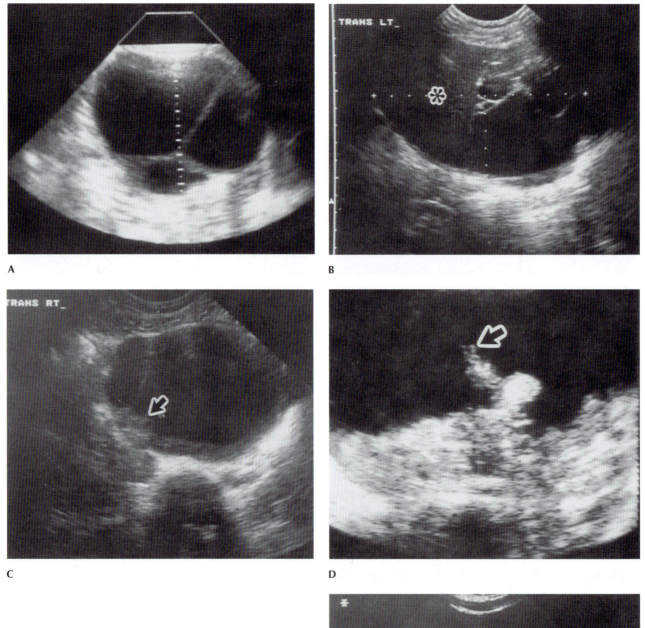

A

B

C

D

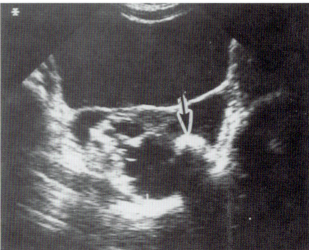

E

FIGURE 5-4 Septated cystic masses. **(A)** Transverse TAS showing cystic mass containing multiple thin internal septations, representing mucinous cystadenoma. **(B)** Transverse TAS showing septated mass with echogenic material (*) in upper loculated area. The echogenic material was mucin within this mucinous cystadenoma. **(C)** Malignancy was suspected due to thickened septation (*arrow*) within this mucinous cystadenocarcinoma. **(D)** Papillary projections (*arrow*) were found within this malignant teratoma. **(E)** Transverse TAS of complex predominantly cystic right-adnexal mass with calcific focus (*arrow*) arising from tooth within this dermoid cyst. *(Figure continued.)*

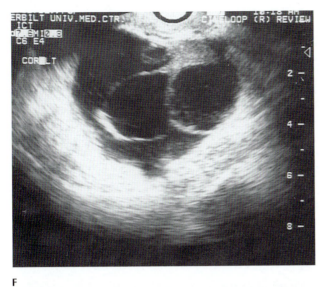

F

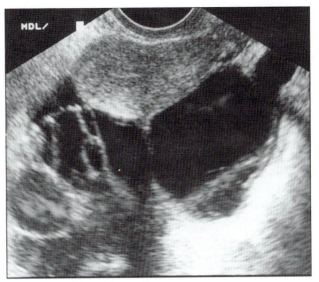

G

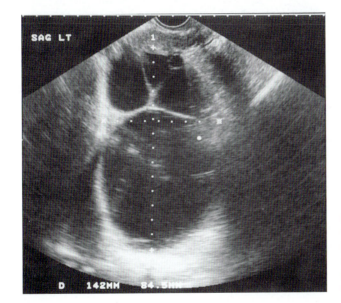

H

FIGURE 5-4 *(continued)* **(F)** TVS of a pelvic mass in a woman with a renal transplant. This was found to represent a luteal cyst with fluid surrounding adhesion. Sagittal **(G)** and axial **(H)** TVS showing a multiloculated septated cystic mass with focal wall thickening. This represented a mucinous cystadenoma with one locule containing thick mucinous material.

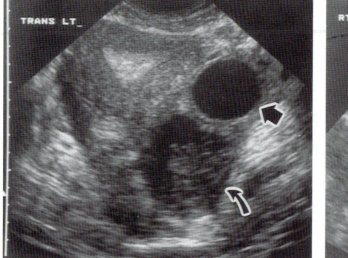

A

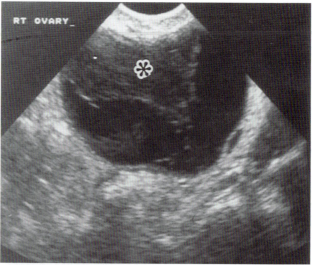

B

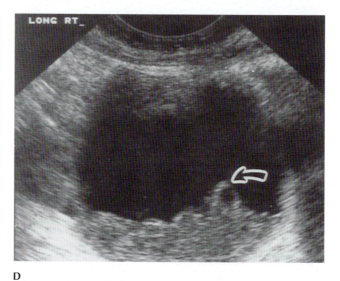

C

D

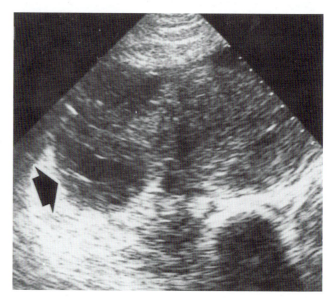

E

FIGURE 5-5 Complex predominantly cystic masses. **(A)** TVS of endometrioma (*curved arrow*) that contained echogenic clot located adjacent to mature follicle (*straight arrow*). **(B)** TVS of tuboovarian abscess. Abscess cavity was surrounded by ovarian tissue (*). **(C)** TVS of hemorrhagic corpus luteum cyst with torsed left ovary. **(D)** TVS of a complex predominantly cystic mass with an irregular solid area and some papillary excrescences (*arrow*). This was a metastasis from a gastrointestinal tract primary tumor. **(E)** Transverse TAS showing cystic right-adnexal mass with septations or strands (*arrow*), representing an appendiceal abscess in a postpartum patient. *(Figure continued.)*

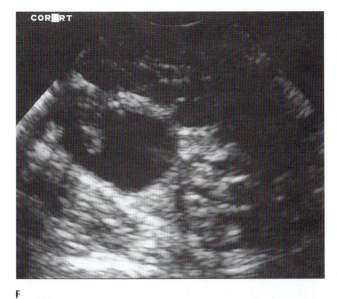

F

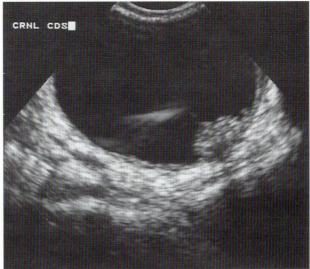

G

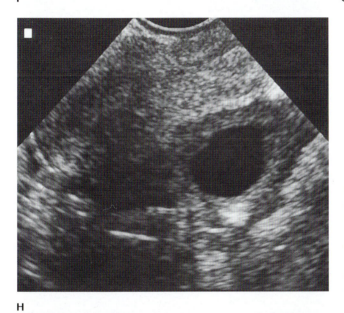

H

FIGURE 5-5 *(continued)* **(F)** TVS of a cystic mass with papillary projection. This represents a cystadenofibroma. The papillae had fibrous and glandular elements. **(G)** TVS of a cystic mass with a papillary excrescence. This was ovarian carcinoma. **(H)** TVS of cystic mass with an irregular wall. This was ovarian cancer. **(I, J)** TVS-guided aspiration of a tubo-ovarian abscess. The patient's fever defervesced after the procedure. The abscess was completely aspirated. *(Figure continued.)*

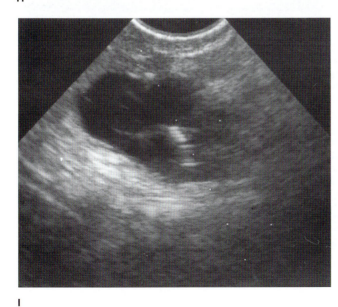

I

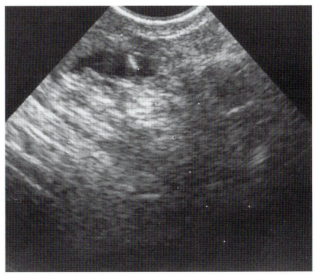

J

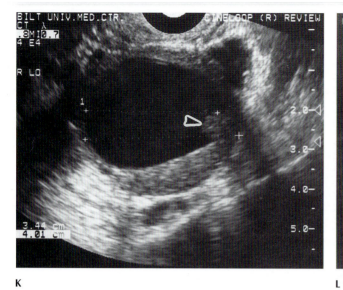

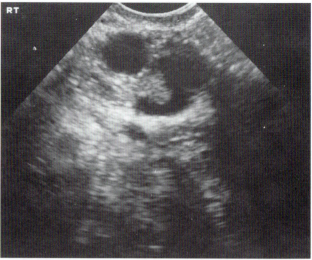

K

L

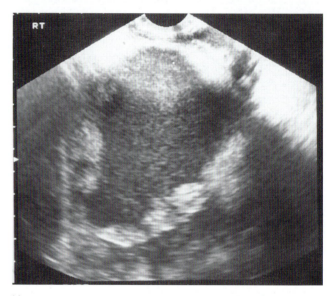

M

FIGURE 5-5 (K) Cystic mass with small focus of solid tissue morphologically similar to a papillary excrescence (*arrowhead*). This mass was benign. **(L)** TVS of a right ovary that contains two cystic masses; one has a papillary excrescence. This was a border-line ovarian cancer adjacent to a mature follicle. **(M)** TVS of a cystic mass with a thick and irregular wall. This was an ovarian carcinoma.

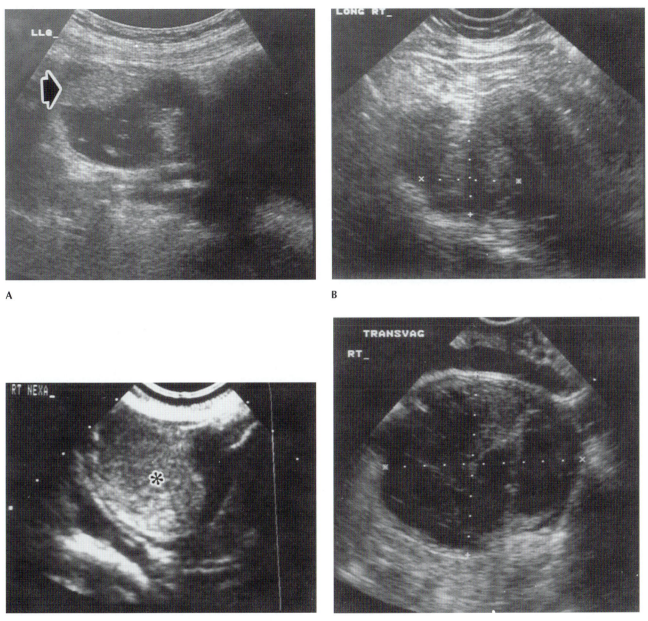

A **B**

C **D**

FIGURE 5-6 Complex predominantly solid masses. **(A)** Predominantly solid, complex mass containing a layer of echogenic material (*arrow*) arising from sebum within this dermoid cyst. **(B)** TVS of a granulosa cell tumor. **(C)** TVS of a dermoid cyst with layer of echogenic sebum. **(D)** TVS of hemorrhagic ovarian cyst containing irregular solid area corresponding to displaced hemorrhagic ovarian tissue surrounding area of hemorrhage. *(Figure continued.)*

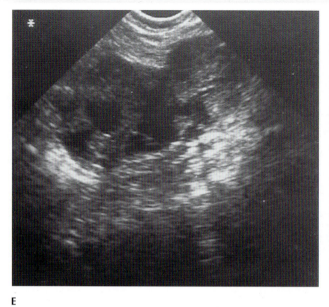

E

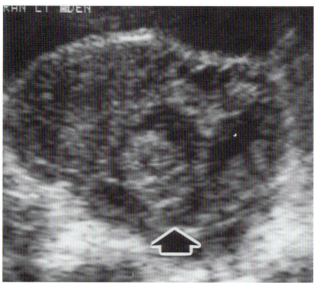

F

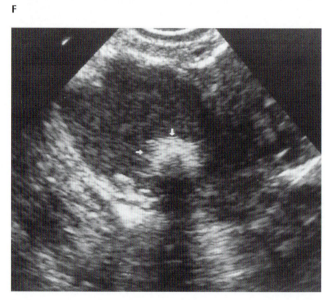

G

FIGURE 5-6 *(continued)* **(E)** Longitudinal TAS of ovarian cyst-adenocarcinoma containing irregular solid areas. **(F)** Magnified transverse TAS of cul-de-sac hemorrhage (*arrow*) resulting from ruptured ectopic pregnancy. **(G)** TVS of dermoid cyst showing typical echogenic hairball (*arrows*).

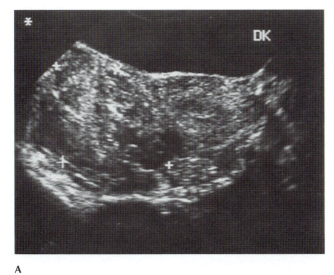

A

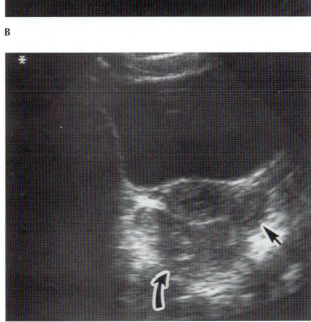

B

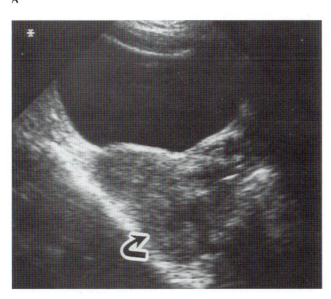

C

D

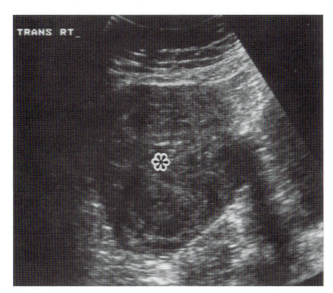

E

FIGURE 5-7 Solid masses. **(A)** Transverse TAS showing enlarged right ovary (*between cursors*) with echogenic areas consistent with hemorrhage due to ovarian rupture. **(B)** Same patient as in **A**, showing intraperitoneal fluid representing blood from ruptured ovary. **(C)** Longitudinal TAS demonstrating solid mass (*arrow*) in cul-de-sac arising from torsed right ovary. **(D)** Transverse TAS of same patient as in **C**, showing that left ovary (*straight arrow*) is normal in size and adjacent to torsed right ovary (*curved arrow*). **(E)** Interligamentous fibroid appearing as solid pelvic mass. *(Figure continued.)*

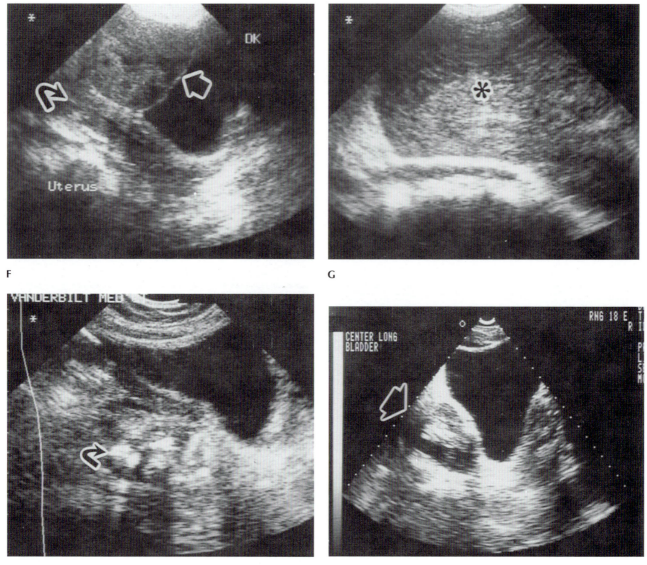

FIGURE 5-7 *(continued)* (F) Myxomatous uterine tumor (*large arrow*) arising from uterine fundus (*curved arrow*). **(G)** Same tumor as in **F**. Ultrasound shows extent of tumor (*), which occupies entire abdomen. **(H)** TAS of a solid pelvic mass with calcifications (*arrow*) in elderly patient. A cystadenofibroma with calcification was found at surgery. **(I)** Longitudinal TAS of pelvic kidney (*arrow*). Pelvocalyceal system accounts for central echogenicity. *(Figure continued.)*

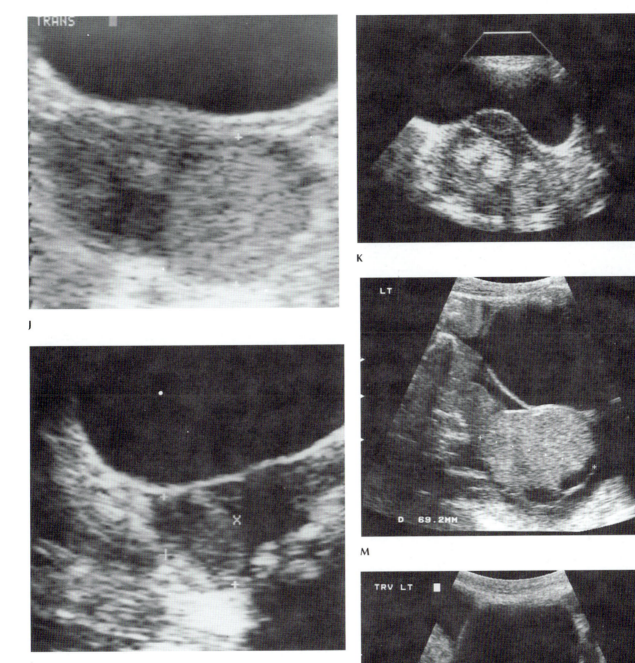

FIGURE 5-7 *(continued)* **(J)** Magnified transverse TAS showing solid left-adnexal mass (*between cursors*), which represents a hemorrhagic corpus luteum cyst. **(K)** Longitudinal TAS of solid teratoma with calcified areas. **(L)** Magnified TAS of solid mass (*between +'s*) representing hemorrhagic corpus luteum cyst. **(M, N)** Sagittal **(M)** and transverse **(N)** TAS showing a 5 × 7 cm solid mass associated with ascites. This was ovarian cancer. *(Figure continued.)*

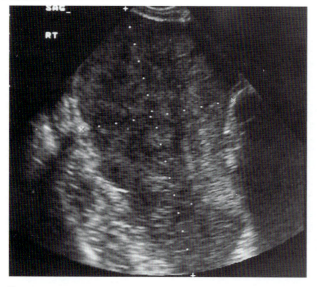

O

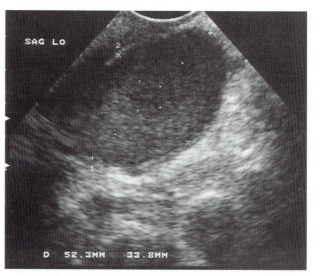

P

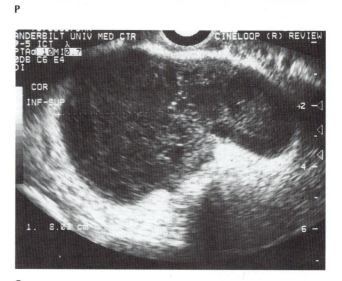

Q

FIGURE 5-7 *(continued)* **(O)** TVS of large solid tumor representing a dysgerminoma. **(P)** TVS of endometrioma showing "ground-glass" texture arising from organized hemorrhage. **(Q)** TVS of pelvic hematoma status, after hysterectomy. The hematoma contains areas of different degrees of organization accounting for its irregular internal texture.

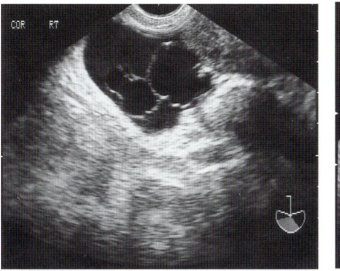

A

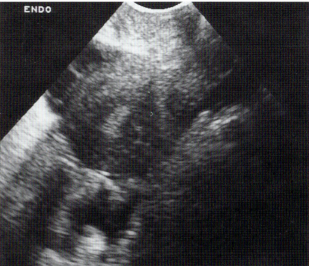

B

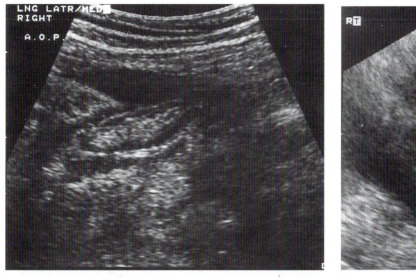

C

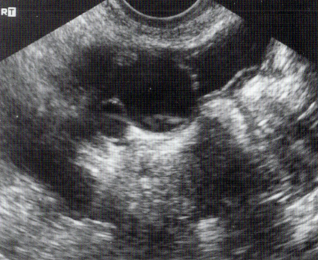

D

FIGURE 5-8 Miscellaneous conditions. **(A)** TVS of loculated fluid with peritoneal adhesions that mimic the appearance of a cystadenoma. TVS **(B)** and TAS **(C)** of a patient presenting with right lower quadrant pain. The TVS shows a normal uterus. Compression TAS demonstrated a thick-walled appendix. This patient had appendicitis at surgery. **(D)** TVS of a patient following bowel surgery showing a peritoneal "pseudocyst" or loculated fluid in the right lower quadrant. *(Figure continued.)*

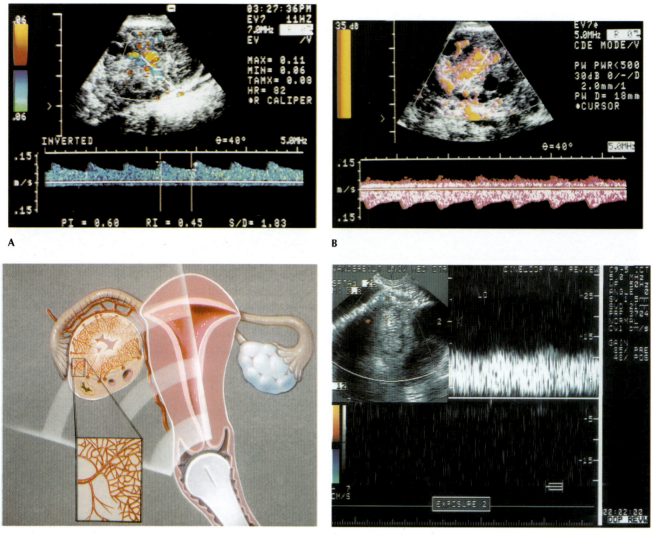

A   **B**

C   **D**

FIGURE 5-9 (A) Frequency transvaginal color Doppler sonogram (TV-CDS) showing low-impedance (pulsatility index of 0.6), low-velocity (maximum systemic velocity = 10 cm/s) flow in the wall of the corpus luteum. **(B)** Amplitude TV-CDS shows more intraparenchymal vascularity than that with frequency-based TV-CDS. **(C)** Disorganized arrangement of vessels with an ovarian tumor. Instead of orderly branching tumor vessels, tumors contain numerous arteriovenous shunts and areas of vessels with stenosis and dilation. The vessels in tumors also tend to be clustered. (*Drawing by Paul Gross, M.S.*) **(D)** TV-CDS of stage I ovarian cancer. Within the papillary excrescence is low-impedance, intermediate-velocity flow. This tumor was found in a young woman who was treated for infertility with ovulation induction. Adjacent to the tumor are two mature follicles.

6 EVALUATION OF PELVIC PAIN

OVERVIEW

- Pelvic pain is one of the common indications for visits to gynecologists.
- There is not always a good correlation between abnormal anatomy/function and pelvic pain.
- The sonographer should use the probe to "probe" for source of pelvic pain.
- Full use of transabdominal sonography (TAS), transvaginal sonography (TVS), and transvaginal color Doppler sonography (TV-CDS) is encouraged in the evaluation of pelvic pain.

ADNEXAL TORSION

- *See Figures 6-1 through 6-6.*
- TV-CDS findings depend on completeness of torsion and chronicity.
- Common associations include:
  - Hemorrhagic ovarian masses
  - Ovarian hyperstimulation
  - Lax ligamentous support
  - Ovarian versus thrombosis
- Typical TVS findings are:
  - Enlarged ovary, which may can contain numerous immature follicles. The ovary may be mildy echogenic due to edema, and have a mildly irregular texture due to the areas of hemorrhage.
  - Cul-de-sac fluid
- TV-CDS findings are variable and depend on the completeness and chronicity of torsion.
  - "Early"—disturbed venous flow; "spiky" arterial waveform
  - "Late"—venous waveform takes on "arterial-oid" shape
  - "Twisted" pedicle can be recognized if there is flow
- Isolated tubal torsion (Fig. 6-7) is most frequently seen in patients who have undergone a bilateral tubal ligation. A fusiform structure with a thick wall and endosalpingeal folds is visible. Flow is absent in the wall.

UTERINE CAUSES

- Adenomyosis has subtle TVS/TV-CDS findings (Fig. 6-8):
  - Irregular bulge in myometrium, referred to as myometrial "cysts"
  - Lack of vascular rim typically seen in fibroids
- Fibroids: more defined area of abnormality than adenomyosis
  - Ischemia/infarction
  - Pedunculated submucosal or subserosal fibroids
  - Vascular rim/pseudocapsule
- Hematometra

ENDOMETRIOSIS

- The findings in "—osis" are subtle in comparison to the distinct TVS findings in "—omas" (Fig. 6-9).
- Adnexal masses with "ground-glass" contents are most diagnostic of endometriomas.
- Punctate echogenicities can be seen within/around the wall and capsule.
- Adnexal immobility is associated with fibrosis.
- Uterosacral ligament deposits and bowel serosal implants are both detectable when there is intraperitoneal fluid; 3D CDS may be helpful to demonstrate their presence.

MISCELLANEOUS CAUSES

PELVIC CONGESTION

- Pelvic congestion is a somewhat controversial cause of pelvic pain because some women with distended parapelvic veins have no pain, while others do.
- Congestion tends to be more common on left since left gonadal vein drains into left renal vein.
- On CDS, distended veins with "to-and-fro" or poor directional flow are visible with Valsalva maneuver (Fig. 6-10).

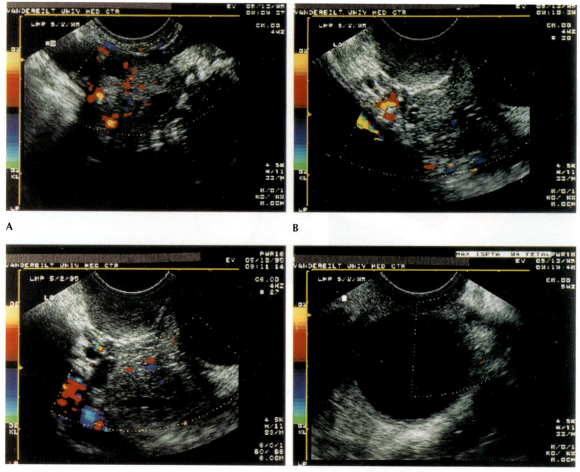

A   B

C   D

FIGURE 6-2 Torsion associated with an adnexal mass. Composite transvaginal color Doppler sono-grams (TV-CDS) of a 28-year-old woman with a 9-hour history of pelvic pain. **(A)** Long axis of perfused right ovary. **(B, C)** Long and short axis images of a mildly enlarged left ovary with intra-ovarian flow. **(D)** A 4-cm paraovarian cyst without flow was present adjacent to the left ovary. At surgery, the adnexa was torsed ×6; however, after excision of the paraovarian cyst, the left ovary was salvaged.

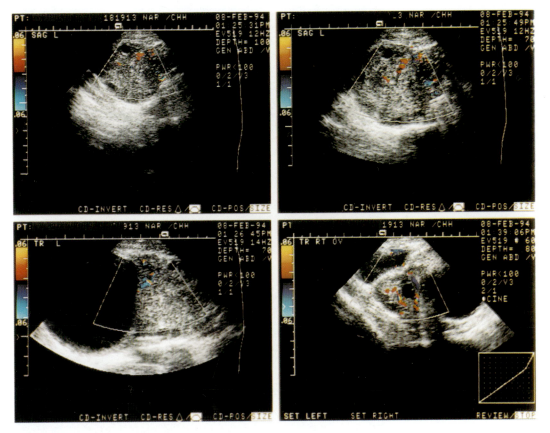

A

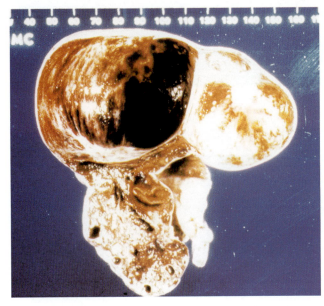

B

FIGURE 6-3 Composite color Doppler sonograms (CDS) of a torsed left ovary containing a cystic mass in a postmenopausal woman found to represent a serous cystadenoma. **(A)** Torsion of the left ovary, which contained the mass, was confirmed at surgery. (*Top left* and *top right*) Enlarged left ovary with flow. (*Bottom left*) Cystic mass arising within the left ovary. (*Bottom right*) Normally perfused right ovary. **(B)** Sectioned specimen showing cystadenoma arising from the left ovary. (*Courtesy of Mary Warner, M.D.*)

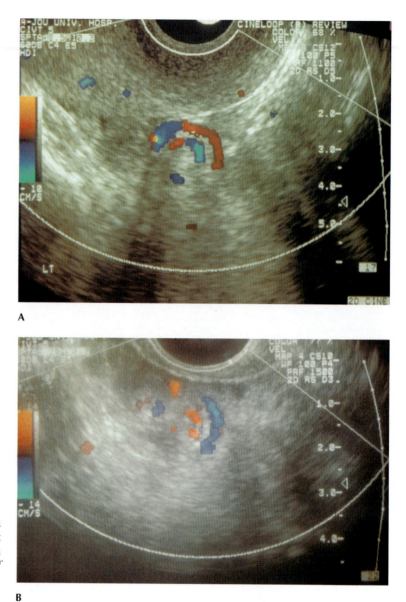

FIGURE 6-4 CDS showing twisted pedicle of a torsed adnexa in two cases (**A**, left ovary; **B**, right ovary) associated with an ovarian teratoma. This sign seems to be specific to adnexal torsion. (*Courtesy of E. Lee, M.D.*)

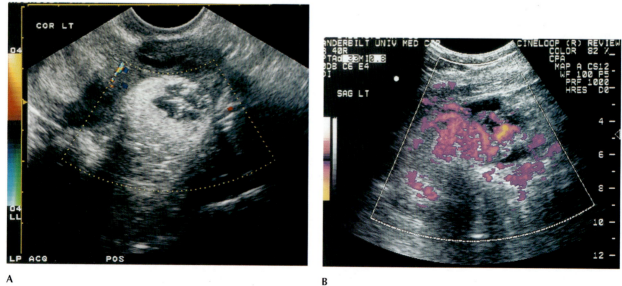

FIGURE 6-5 TV-CDS of torsed and de-torsed ovary containing a dermoid cyst. (**A**) The initial TV-CDS shows no flow within the echogenic mass within the left ovary. (**B**) After surgical de-torsion, this amplitude TV-CDS showed flow.

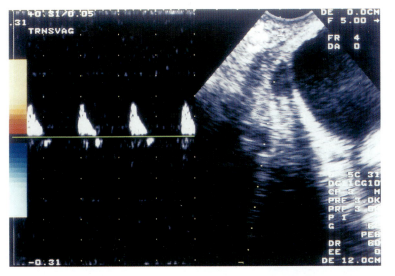

A

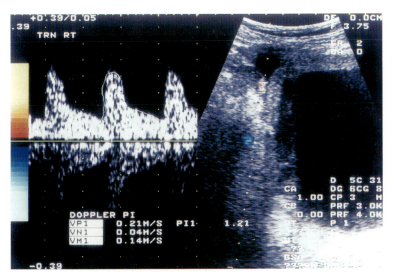

B

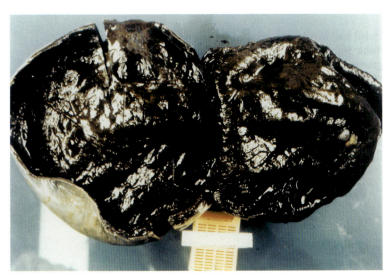

C

FIGURE 6-6 Torsed hemorrhagic cyst in a patient several years following hysterectomy. **(A)** The adnexal branch of the uterine artery shows absent diastolic flow. **(B)** In other areas around the cyst, there is normal arterial flow. **(C)** The resected specimen shows a gangrenous hemorrhagic ovary. The flow was maintained to the right tube, accounting for the normal flow seen in one area.

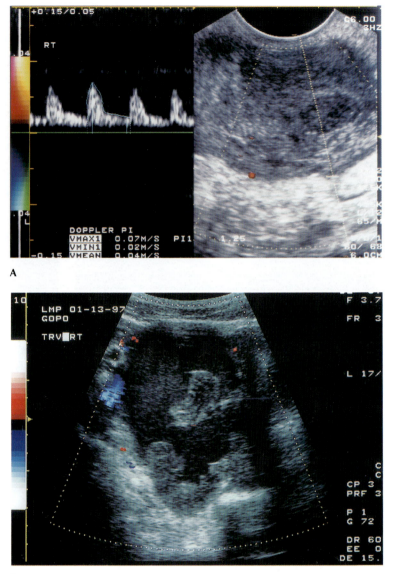

FIGURE 6-9 Endometriomas. **(A)** TV-CDS of a hemorrhagic mass representing an endometrioma containing organized hemorrhage. **(B)** Transabdominal CDS (TA-CDS) of a mass containing solid areas without flow, representing an organized clot within this endometrioma.

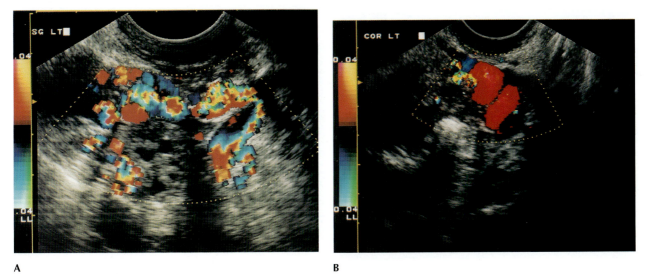

A   B

FIGURE 6-10 TV-CDS of pelvic congestion. **(A)** CDS of distended pelvic veins as seen in long axis in a patient with intermittent pelvic pain. **(B)** TV-CDS showing distended papapelvic veins in an asymptomatic woman.

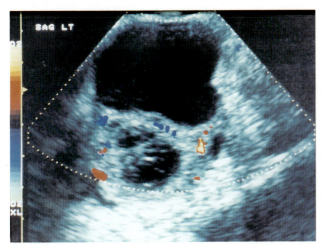

FIGURE 6-11 CDS of an ovarian remnant containing a hemorrhagic corpus luteum.

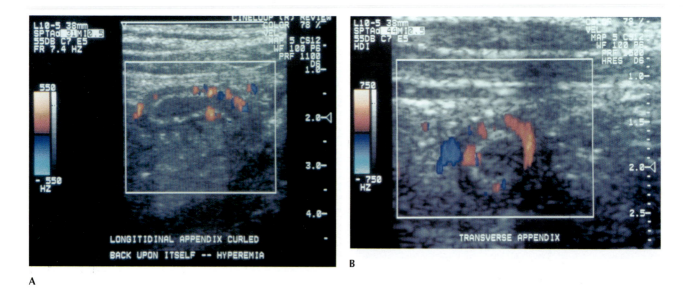

A

B

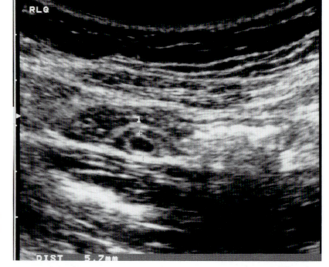

C

FIGURE 6-12 Appendicitis. **(A,B)** TA-CDS of appendicitis showing thickened and hyperemic appendiceal wall in long **(A)** and short **(B)** axes. (*Courtesy of ATL, Inc.*) **(C)** Thickened appendiceal wall (*between cursors*) in a patient with right lower quadrant pain. An unruptured appendix with acute inflammation was found at surgery.

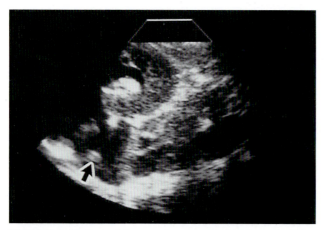

FIGURE 6-13 Coronal image of maternal left kidney showing echogenic focus (*arrow*) with renal pelvis corresponding to renal calculi.

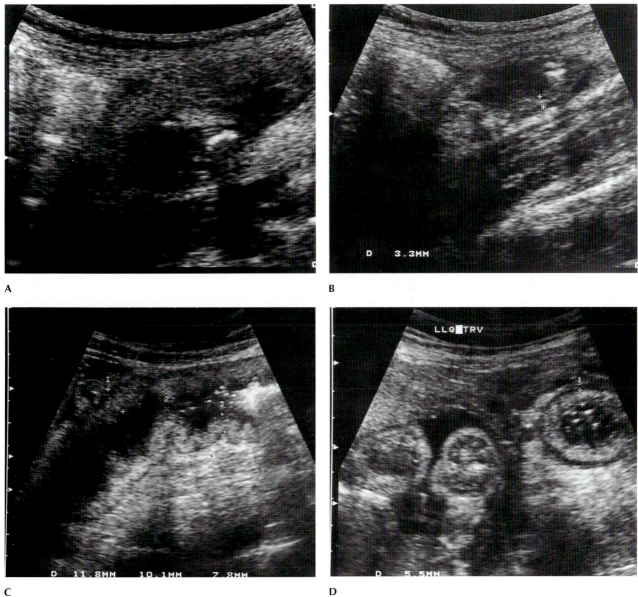

FIGURE 6-14 Maternal bowel disorders. **(A)** Transverse sonogram showing thickened large bowel wall in a patient with pseudomembranous colitis. **(B)** Short-axis image showing thickened bowel wall *(between cursors)* of patient shown in **A**. **(C)** Transverse sonogram showing thickened large bowel wall in a patient with pseudomembranous colitis. **(D)** Short-axis image showing thickened bowel wall *(between +'s)* of patient shown in **C**.

7 MISCELLANEOUS GYNECOLOGIC DISORDERS

INFERTILITY

- Transvaginal sonography (TVS) has multiple roles in the treatment and evaluation of fertility disorders:
  - Assessment of follicular maturity (Fig. 7-1) and abnormalities of ovulation
  - Assessment of endometrial development (Fig. 7-2)
  - Assessment of ovarian/endometrial blood flow
  - Evaluation of tubal patency
  - Detection and evaluation of uterine malformations
  - Guided follicular aspiration
  - Detection of adhesions, submucosal fibroids, and polyps with sonohysterography (SHG)
  - Evaluation of complicated early pregnancy, multifetal pregnancy

FOLLICULAR MONITORING

- Mature follicles measure between 18 and 25 mm.
- Corpora lutea have a crenated border and rim vascularity.
- In induced cycles (Fig. 7-3), multiple follicles are coaxed to mature with clomiphene citrate (Clomid).
- Multiple mature follicles are usually seen with human menopausal gonadotrophin (Pergonal).
- Multiple follicles typically have various levels of maturity.

OVARIAN HYPERSTIMULATION SYNDROME

- Ovarian hyperstimulation syndrome (Fig. 7-4) can occur as hypersensitivity to ovulation induction.
- Some patients may be pregnant when they become symptomatic.
- There is acute swelling of the ovaries.
- There is ascites and electrolyte imbalance.
- Ovaries are usually enlarged and contain numerous hydropic follicles
- Ascites is due to "third spacing."
- The enlarged ovaries may torse.

ENDOMETRIAL ASSESSMENT

- Midcycle endometrium has a multilayered pattern with an echogenic basal layer.
- Outer interface and functionalis layer are hypoechoic.
- Bilayer thickness should be between 5 and 8 mm in midcycle.
- Luteal endometrium has spiral vascularity.

TUBAL PATENCY

- *See Figures 7-5 and 7-6.*
- SHG is performed with a balloon-tipped catheter to block antegrade flow of instilled saline and encourage antegrade flow through tubes.
- To best delineate the tube, line up the cornual endometrium with the ovary, and watch for "sparking" of fluid. Use positive contrast if the portion of the study using saline is inconclusive.

UTERINE MALFORMATIONS

- TVS can identify the endometrium, especially in the luteal phase.
- 3D sonography (3D US) is very useful in characterizing uterine shape, especially evaluation of uterine fundus for notch seen in bicornuate, not in septated uterus (Fig. 7-7).
- Magnetic resonance imaging (MRI) is an excellent secondary modality for evaluation of uterine shape.

GUIDED FOLLICULAR ASPIRATION

- Use needle guide attached to probe (Fig. 7-8).
- Line up target and projected path.
- Avoid parauterine vessels.

DETECTION OF SUBMUCOSAL FIBROIDS, POLYPS, AND ADHESIONS

- SHG (Fig. 7-9) can detect polyps and submucosal fibroids, and determine their extension into lumen and

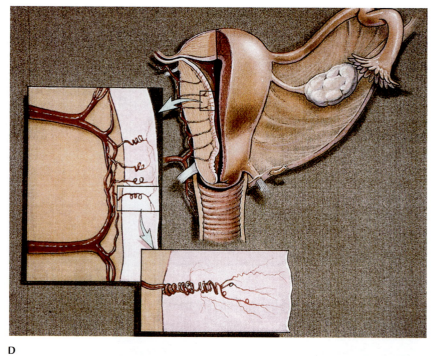

D

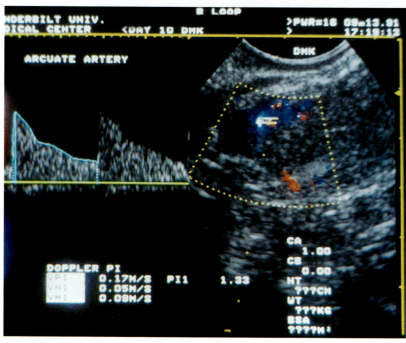

FIGURE 7-2 *(continued)* **(D)** Diagram of the uterine arterial tree. The arcuate arterioles branch into radial, which course across the myometrium ending in the spiral arteries within the endometrium. **(E)** TV-CDS of arcuate artery flow at day 10. *(Figure continued.)*

E

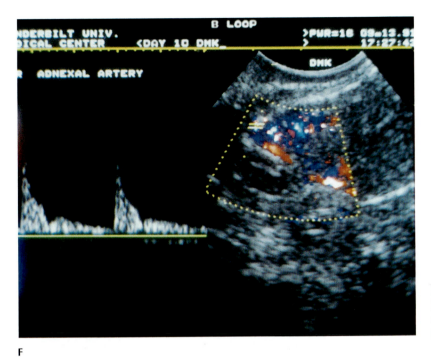

F

FIGURE 7-2 *(continued)* **(F)** Same patient as in **E** showing the adnexal branch of the uterine artery. Note the area of flow within the myometrium.

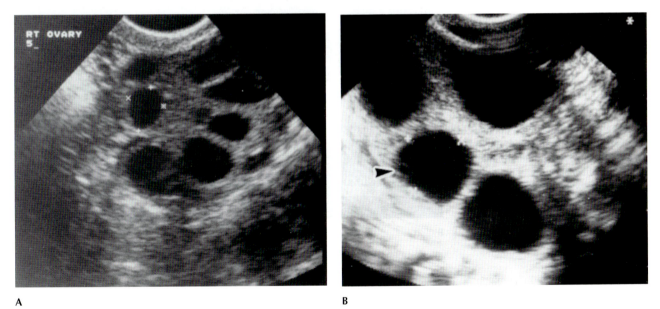

A   B

FIGURE 7-3 Follicular monitoring in induced cycles. **(A)** TVS of multiple follicles in various developmental stages in a patient undergoing induction of ovulation with human menopausal gonadotropin. **(B)** Magnified TVS in a patient undergoing induction of ovulation with clomiphene citrate. Along the edge of the follicle, denoted by cursors, the cumulus can be identified (*arrowhead*).

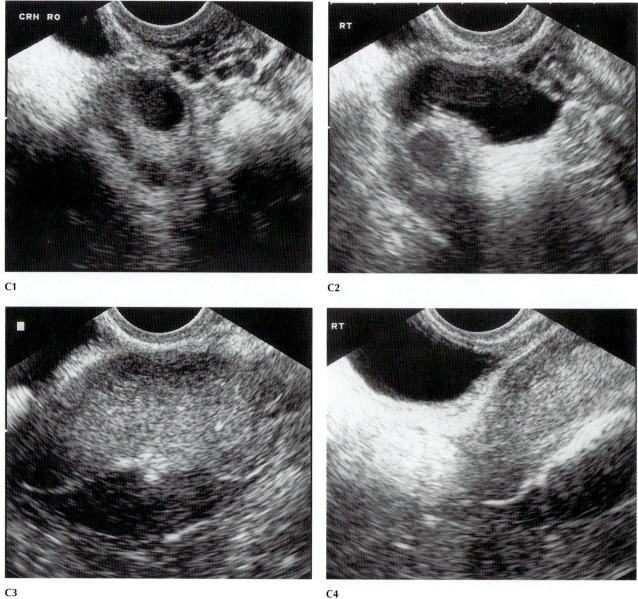

C1

C2

C3

C4

FIGURE 7-6 *(continued)* **(C)** Bilaterally patent tubes. **(C1)** Before sonohysterography (SHG), the right ovary contains a nearly mature follicle. **(C2)** After SHG, saline pools around the right ovary. **(C3)** "Catfish" configuration of the tubal ostia as depicted in transverse sections shows contrast in both proximal tubes. **(C4)** The right tube could be followed into its interstitial portion. *(Figure continued.)*

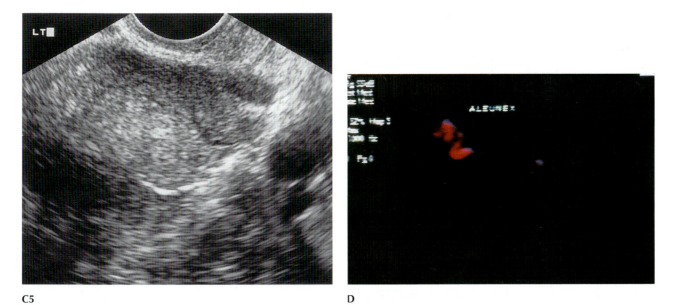

C5   D

FIGURE 7-6 *(continued)* **(C5)** Same as **C4**, showing the proximal left tube. **(D)** Three-dimensional CDS (3D CDS) of normal tube obtained during Albunex instillation using harmonic imaging.

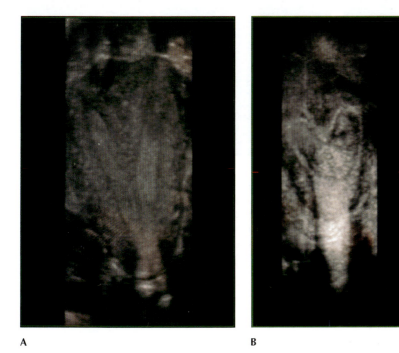

A   B

FIGURE 7-7 Three-dimensional sonography (3D US) of uterine malformation. **(A)** 3D US in mid-coronal plane showing two endometrial cavities and smooth configuration of uterine fundus, an indication of septated uterus. **(B)** Bicornuate uterus with hematometra within heart-shaped lumen.

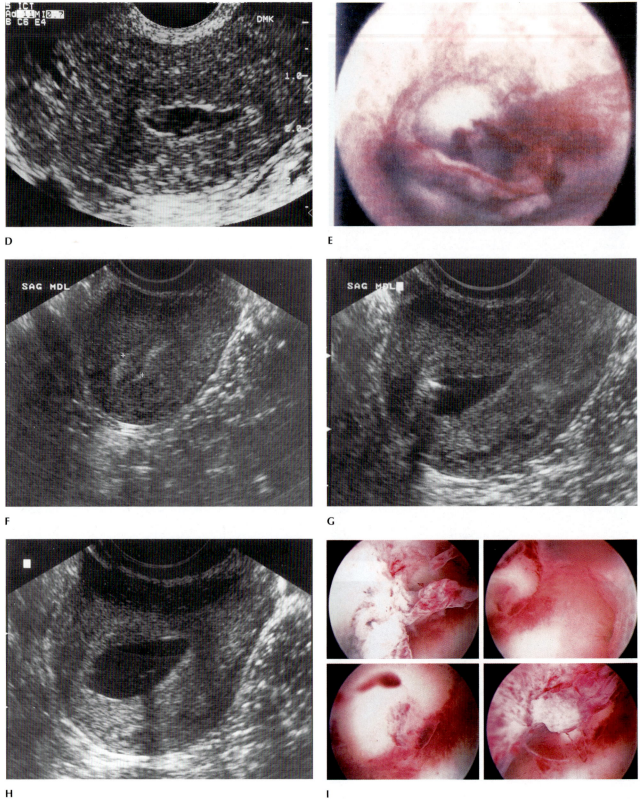

D

E

F

G

H

I

FIGURE 7-9 *(continued)* **(D)** SHG showing adhesion appearing as echogenic interface crossing the lumen. **(E)** Hysteroscopic view of adhesion in patient in **D**. *(Courtesy of Ester Eisenberg, M.D.)* **(F)** Initial TVS of patient before SHG. The endometrium *(between cursors)* is slightly irregular in this patient who had a history of several miscarriages. **(G)** After saline distention, there is mild irregularity of the endometrium in the fundus. **(H)** Same patient as in **F** and **G**, with more distention confirming the slightly irregular fundal endometrium. **(I)** Hysteroscopic images of patient in **F–H**, showing "heaped up" endometrium fundal area. *(Figure continued.)*

146

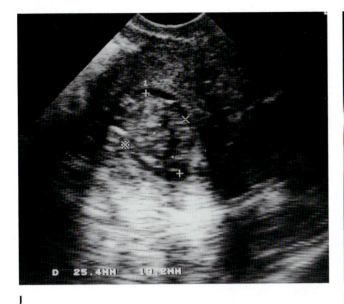

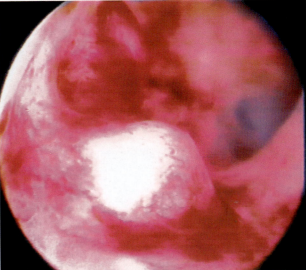

J

K

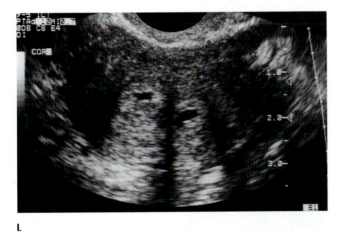

L

FIGURE 7-9 *(continued)* **(J)** SHG showing a submucosal fibroid (*between cursors*). **(K)** Hysteroscopic view of patient in **J** showing submucosal fibroid. **(L)** SHG showing double lumina of bicornuate uterus. Note the fundal cleft. **(M)** SHG in an infertility patient showing a fundal polyp. **(N, O)** TV-CDS of patient in **M** showing vascular pedicle of the polyp in long **(N)** and short **(O)** axes.

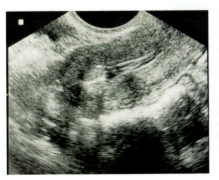

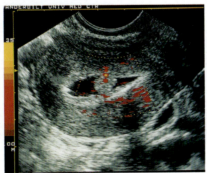

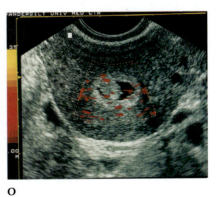

M

N

O

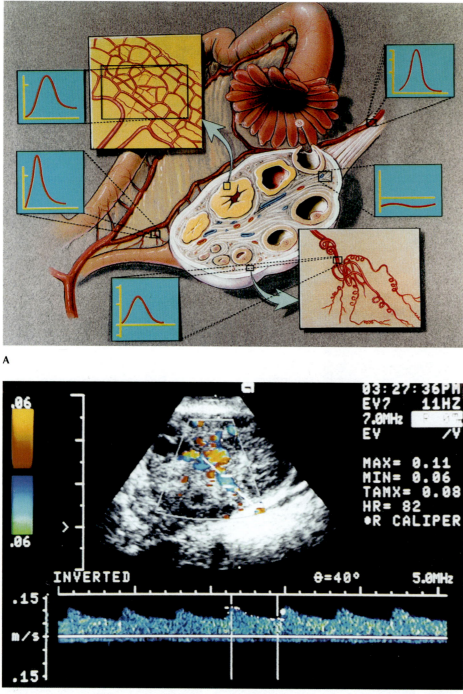

A

B

FIGURE 7-10 Principles of tumor detection with TV-CDS. **(A)** Diagram of typical ovarian arterial waveforms. The waveform will depend on whether it is obtained in an area of folliculogenesis or corpus luteum. In areas devoid of follicles the resistance is high; around a corpus luteum with its "vascular arcade" the waveforms show low-resistance, high-diastolic flow. (*Drawing by Paul Gross, M.S.*) **(B)** Normal TV-CDS showing low-impedance flow in an intraovarian arteriole surrounding a functioning corpus luteum. *(Figure continued.)*

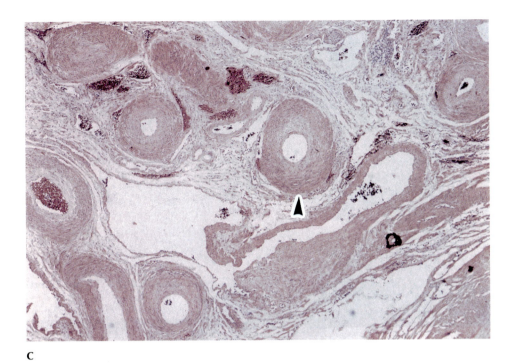

C

D

FIGURE 7-10 *(continued)* **(C)** Photomicrograph shows histologic specimen of normal ovary showing muscular media *(arrowhead)* within a normal intraovarian arteriole. **(D)** Diagram showing early-stage ovarian tumor. The vessels have an irregular branching pattern. *(Drawing by Paul Gross, MS.)* *(Figure continued.)*

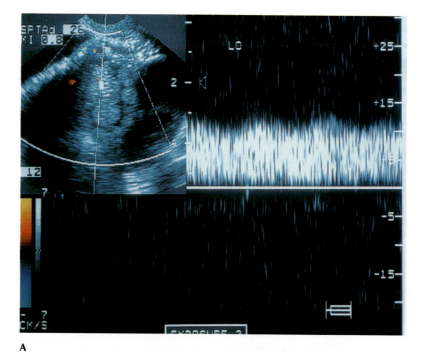

A

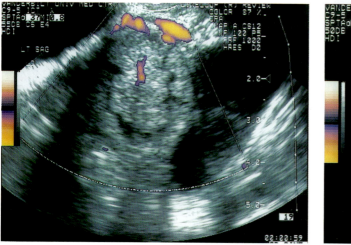

B

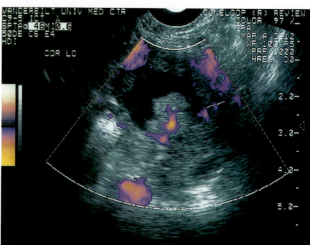

C

FIGURE 7-12 Increased flow within a papillary excrescence within an ovary that contained two mature follicles in a 39-year-old patient undergoing ovulation induction. This was stage II ovarian cancer. **(A)** TV-CDS shows low-impedance flow within papillary excrescence. There are two mature follicles within this ovary. **(B, C)** Amplitude TV-CDS shows flow within the papillary excrescence on long **(B)** and short **(C)** axes. **(D)** Photomicrograph shows increased number of vessels within the papillary excrescence.

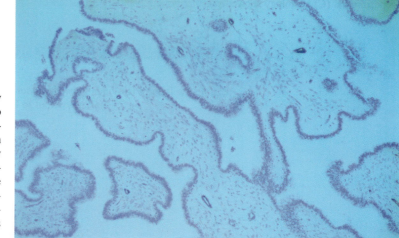

D

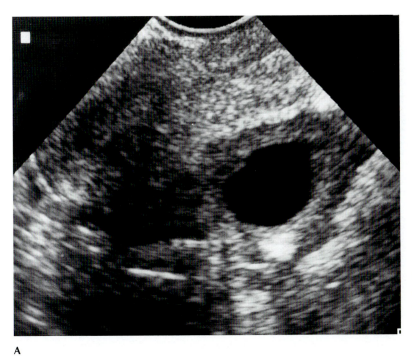

A

FIGURE 7-13 Irregular wall in a mostly cystic ovary of a 43-year-old woman. This was stage II ovarian cancer. **(A)** TVS shows irregularity in the wall of a cystic mass within the left ovary. *(Figure continued.)*

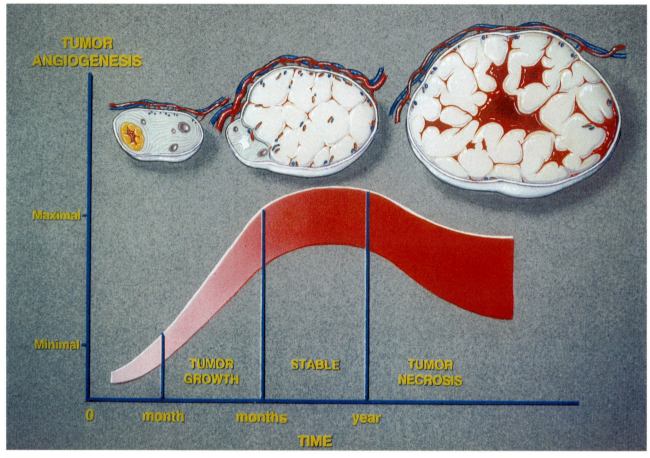

FIGURE 7-14 Diagram showing vascularity relative to tumor growth. (*Drawing by Paul Gross, M.S.*) In early stages, the tumor is very vascular. As the tumor enlarges, the vascularity may decrease in areas of tumor infarction due to outgrowing the blood supply.

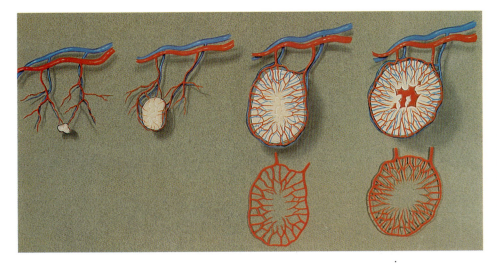

FIGURE 7-15 Tumor angiogenesis. In order for a tumor to enlarge, it incites new blood vessels to develop from the host. The vascular network is tenuous, with areas of focal ischemia. The vascular network has many arteriovenous communications, which results in a low-impedance vascular network.

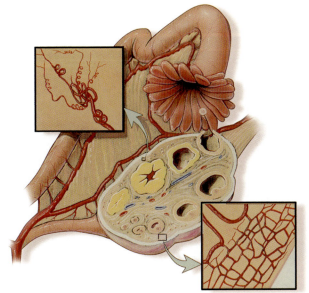

FIGURE 7-16 Ovarian vasculature. Within the ovary, the vessels have a variety of appearances, depending on the presence of a functioning corpus luteum. In the wall of a functioning corpus luteum, there is low-impedance flow.

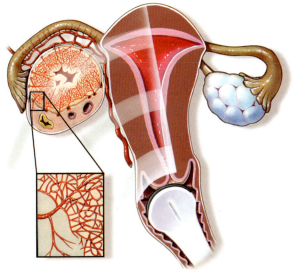

FIGURE 7-17 In ovarian tumors, there is a tenuous vascular network, with clusters of abnormal vessels.

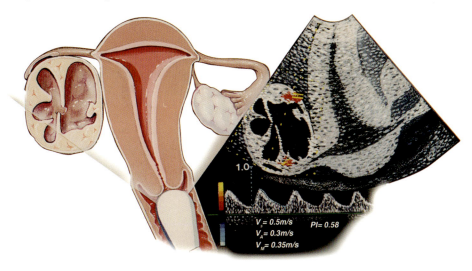

FIGURE 7-18 With triplex TV-CDS, these areas of abnormal vessels demonstrate low-impedance flow.

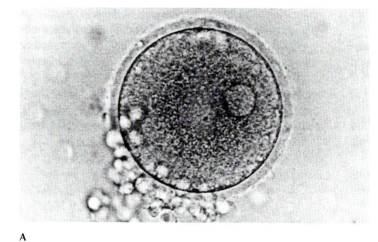

A

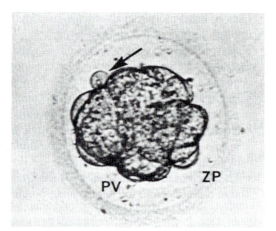

B

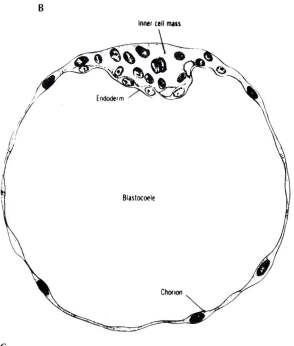

C

FIGURE 8-1 Embryonic/early fetal development. **(A)** Human oocyte in process of fertilization (× 420). **(B)** A preimplantation baboon embryo (similar to the human) as the morula is transforming into a blastocyst. Arrow, column segmentation cavity; PV, perivitelline space; ZP, zona pellucida. **(C)** Line drawing of blastocyst showing early inner cell mass and trophoblast. (*Reprinted with permission from Davies J. Human Developmental Anatomy. New York: Ronald, 1963.*) **(D)** Section of 11-day human embryo showing cellular and syncytial trophoblast. (*Reprinted with permission from Arey B. Developmental Anatomy. Philadelphia: Saunders, 1962.*) *(Figure continued.)*

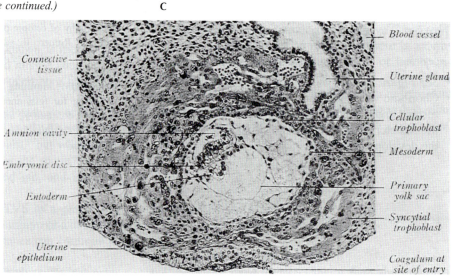

D

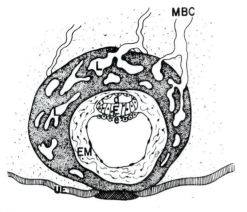

E

F

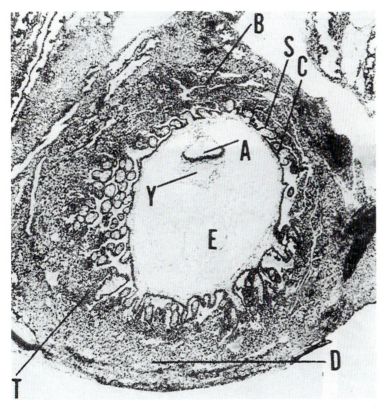

G

FIGURE 8-1 *(continued)* **(E)** 12-day implanted embryo. a, Amnion and amniotic cavity; E, embryonic ectoderm; e, embryonic entoderm; EM, extraembryonic mesenchyme; L, maternal blood lacuna in the trophoblast; UE, uterine epithelium; MBC, maternal blood circulation. (*Redrawn by Panigel. In: Grasse, ed.* Traite de Zoologie. *Paris: Masson, 1976. Reprinted with permission from Hertig and Rock and from Starck.*) **(F)** Cross section of early human placenta that demonstrates portions of the villous tree and stem villi anchored to the decidua basalis. (*Reprinted with permission from Davies J.* Human Developmental Anatomy. *New York: Ronald, 1963.*) **(G)** Cross section through an early (16-day) gestational sac. B, Decidual basalis; D, decidual capsularis; T, cytotrophoblast; C, chorion; S, secondary villus; A, amnion; Y, yolk sac; E, exocoelomic cavity. (*Reprinted with permission from Gruenwald P.* The Placenta. *Baltimore: University Park Press, 1975.*) *(Figure continued.)*

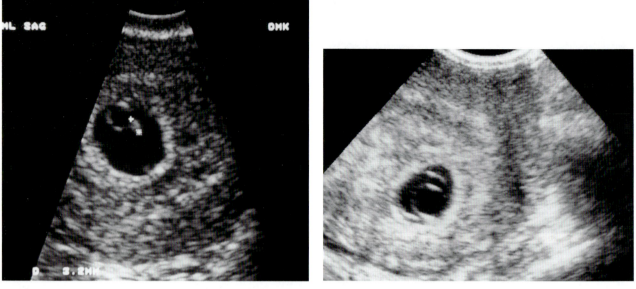

F   G

FIGURE 8-3 *(continued)* **(F)** TVS showing embryo/yolk sac complex. The embryo is 3 mm in size, and heart motion was seen. **(G)** TVS of "deflated" gestational sac with enlarged yolk sac but no definite embryo. This is consistent with embryonic demise.

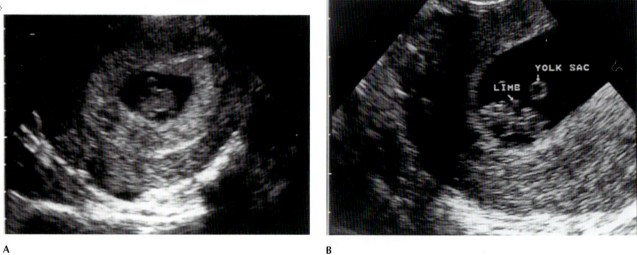

A   B

FIGURE 8-4 Normal 7- to 8-week IUP. **(A)** TVS of 8-mm embryo with a yolk sac adjacent to embryo. **(B)** Ten-millimeter embryo demonstrating limb and yolk sac. *(Figure continued.)*

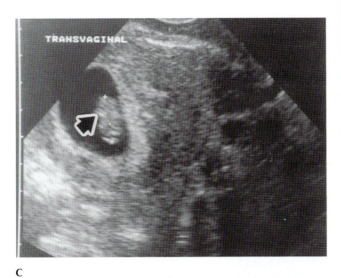

C

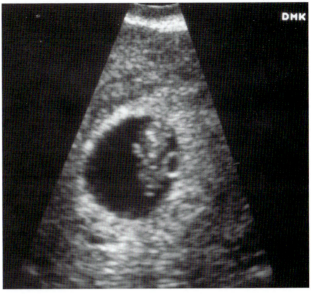

D

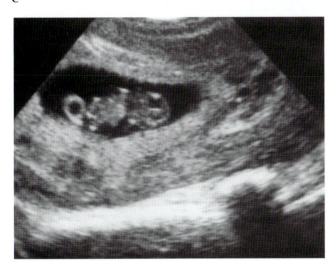

E

FIGURE 8-4 *(continued)* **(C)** TVS of 8-week embryo in coronal plane, demonstrating early ossification of clavicle (*arrow*). **(D)** Seven-week embryo with adjacent yolk sac. The arm buds are seen. **(E)** Eight-to-nine-week pregnancy showing the developing head (rhombencephalon). The choriodecidua now is intact.

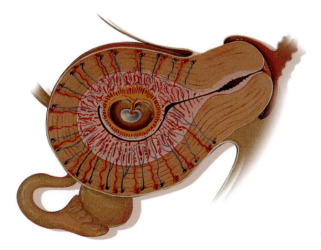

FIGURE 8-5 The vessels within the uterus in early pregnancy. Arcuate vessels traverse the myometrium as radial branches that supply the deciduas capsularis and vera. Color should also be emanating from the fetal heart.

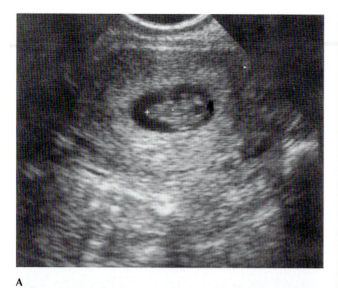

A

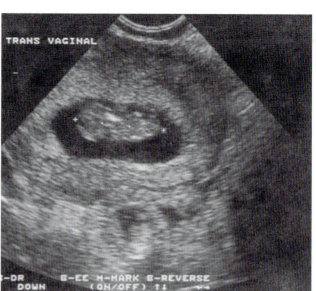

TRANS VAGINAL

B

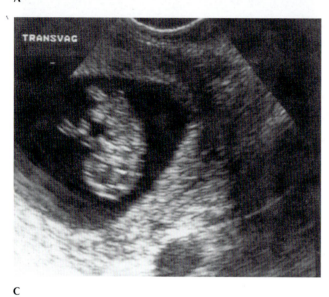

TRANSVAG

C

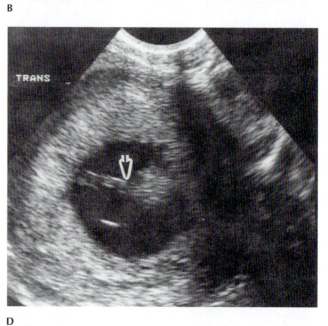

TRANS

D

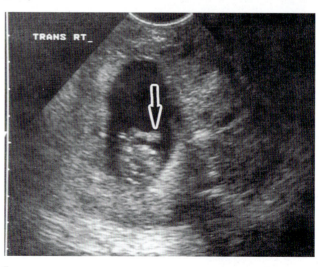

TRANS RT

E

FIGURE 8-6 Normal fetal anatomy. **(A)** TVS of 17-mm embryo demonstrating prominent cystic area of brain corresponding to rhombencephalon. **(B)** TVS of 28-mm fetus. **(C)** TVS of 10-week fetus demonstrating arms and legs. **(D)** Transverse view of same fetus showing umbilical cord insertion within some physiologic herniation of bowel into base of umbilical cord. **(E)** TVS showing hands on or near face of 11-week fetus. *(Figure continued.)*

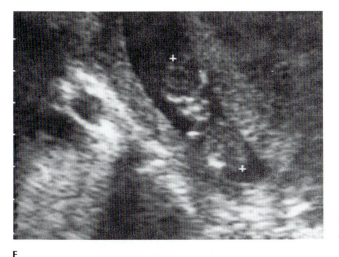

F

FIGURE 8-6 *(continued)* **(F)** TAS of 11-week fetus *(between cursors)*.

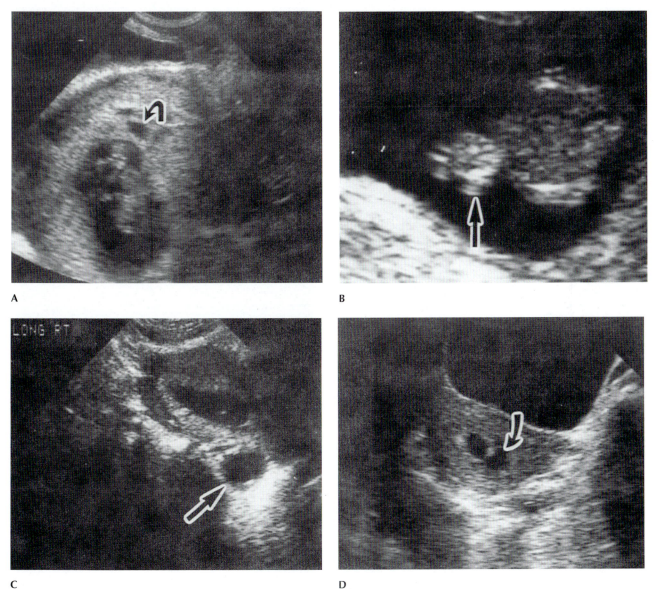

A

B

C

D

FIGURE 8-7 Other normal features. **(A)** Hypoechoic lacunae *(curved arrow)* around decidua basalis of 10-week IUP. **(B)** Magnified TVS of 11-week fetus with bowel herniated into base of cord. **(C)** TAS of corpus luteum cyst of pregnancy. **(D)** TAS showing unoccupied lumen *(curved arrow)* at 6 weeks. *(Figure continued.)*

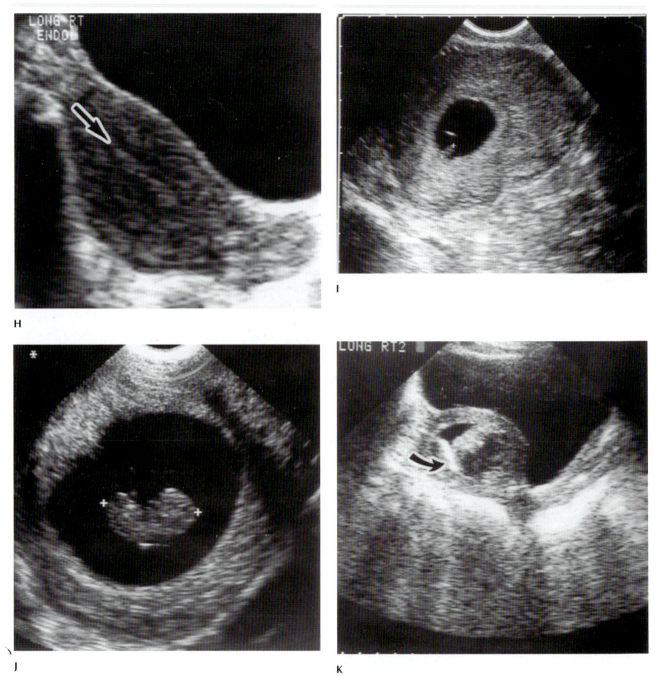

FIGURE 8-9 *(continued)* **(H)** TAS of completed abortion. Note thinness and regularity of endometrial interfaces *(arrow)*. **(I)** TVS of embryonic demise at 6 weeks. No heart activity was detected. **(J)** TVS of fetal demise at 9 weeks. No heart motion was detected. **(K)** TAS showing retrochorionic hemorrhage surrounding an IUD *(curved arrow)*. The deflated sac is seen inferior to the IUD. *(Figure continued.)*

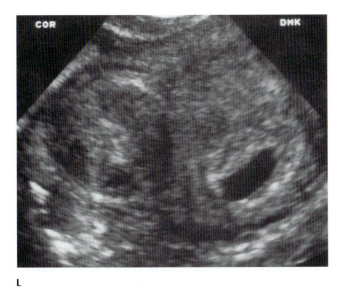

L

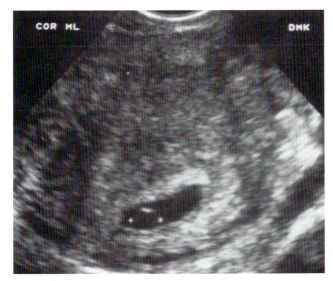

A

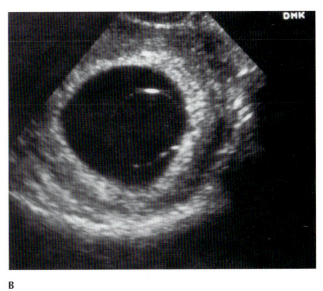

B

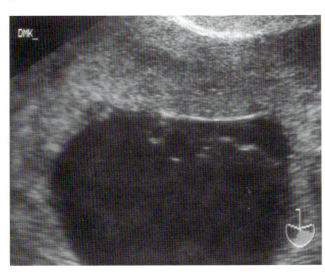

C

FIGURE 8-9 *(continued)* **(L)** TVS showing large fibroid on maternal right and normal gestational sac to the left of midline.

FIGURE 8-10 Gestational sac anomalies. **(A)** Yolk sac within an overall small gestational sac. **(B)** Large gestational sac. The amnion could be seen within the sac but no definite embryo. These are two ends of the spectrum seen in intrauterine fetal demise. **(C)** Vitelline duct leading to a deflated yolk sac. *(Figure continued.)*

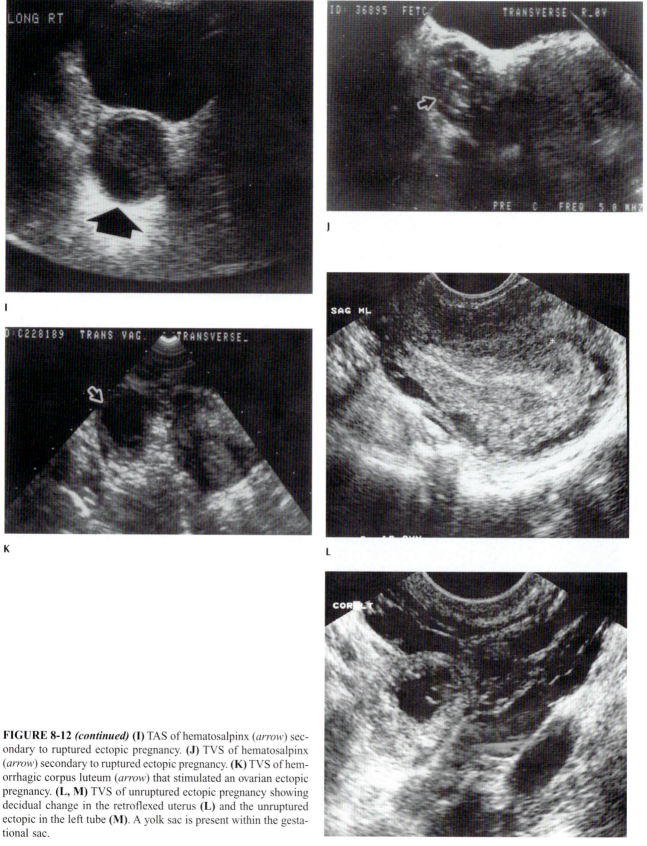

FIGURE 8-12 *(continued)* **(I)** TAS of hematosalpinx *(arrow)* secondary to ruptured ectopic pregnancy. **(J)** TVS of hematosalpinx *(arrow)* secondary to ruptured ectopic pregnancy. **(K)** TVS of hemorrhagic corpus luteum *(arrow)* that stimulated an ovarian ectopic pregnancy. **(L, M)** TVS of unruptured ectopic pregnancy showing decidual change in the retroflexed uterus **(L)** and the unruptured ectopic in the left tube **(M)**. A yolk sac is present within the gestational sac.

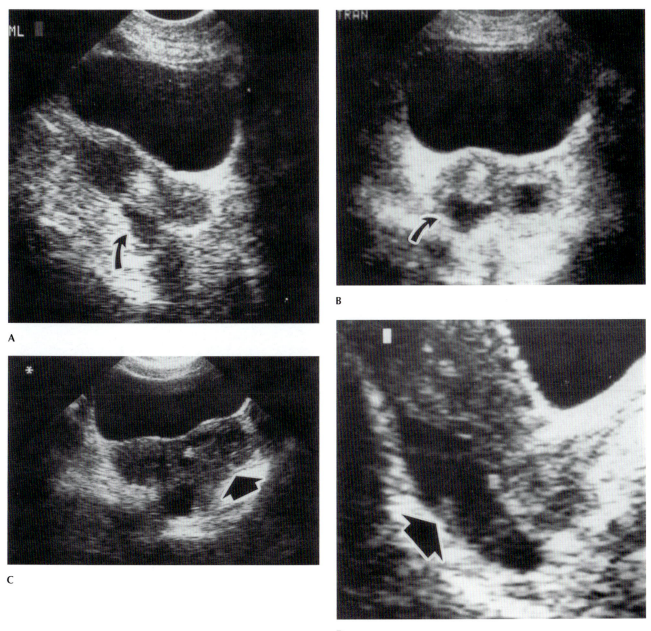

FIGURE 8-13 Ectopic pregnancy: peritoneal findings. **(A)** Longitudinal and **(B)** transverse sonograms of "leaking" left tubal ectopic pregnancy with unclotted cul-de-sac hemorrhage (*curved arrow*). **(C)** Transverse TAS of clotted hemorrhage secondary to chronic ruptured ectopic pregnancy. **(D)** Magnified longitudinal TAS showing partially clotted cul-de-sac hemorrhage (*arrow*) secondary to ruptured ectopic pregnancy. *(Figure continued.)*

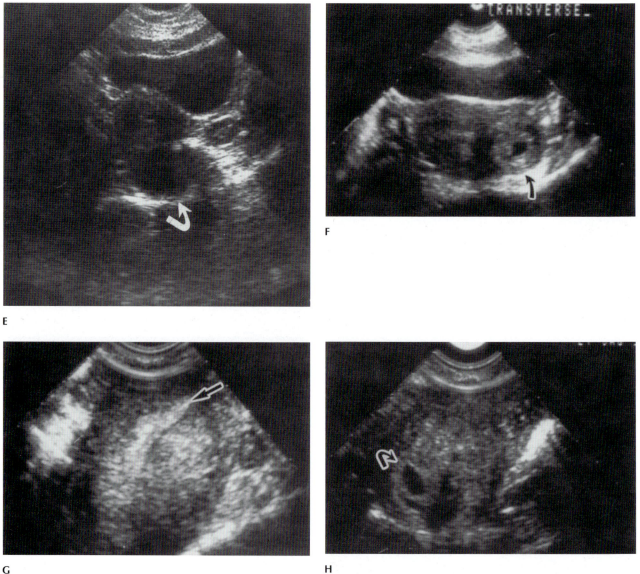

FIGURE 8-15 *(continued)* **(E)** Transverse TAS of patient with cystic adnexal mass and positive pregnancy test. At surgery, ectopic pregnancy was found next to a cystadenoma of left ovary (*curved arrow*). **(F)** Transverse TAS showing eccentrically located gestational sac (*curved arrow*). **(G)** TVS showing thickened endometrium (*arrow*) of nongravid horn of a bicornuate uterus. **(H)** Left horn contained a gestational sac (*curved arrow*). **F** through **H** are from the same patient. *(Figure continued.)*

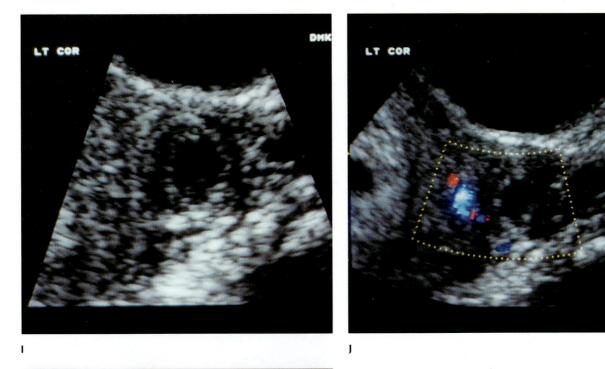

I

J

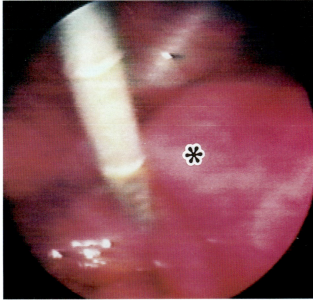

K

FIGURE 8-15 *(continued)* **(I)** Magnified TVS showing a rounded mass near left cornu. **(J)** TV-CDS of same patient in **J** showing rounded mass near left cornu coexisiting with a 6-week intrauterine pregnancy. Only a portion of the intrauterine sac is seen. **(K)** Photograph taken during laparoscopy showing round ligament fibroma (*). *(Courtesy of Barbara Nylander, M.D)*. *(Figure continued.)*

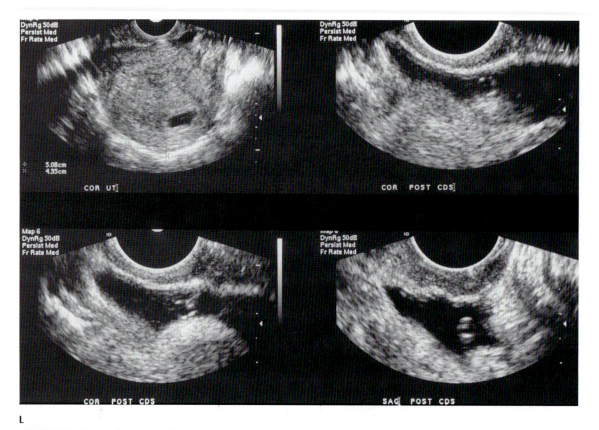

L

FIGURE 8-15 *(continued)* **(L)** Composite TVS showing fluid in cul-de-sac surrounding a rounded structure. This most likely represented a cyst of Morgangi that arose from the frimbriated end of the tube. The presence of fluid surrounding it allowed its sonographic delineation. Initially, a yolk sac was considered, but a cyst of Morgangi was considered possible although not confirmed at surgery, because the patient had an ongoing pregnancy.

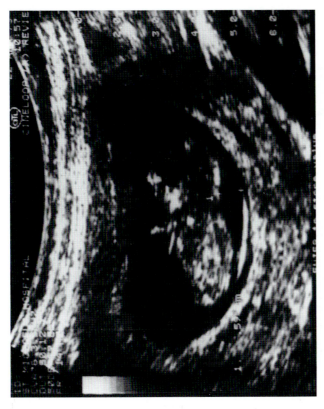

A

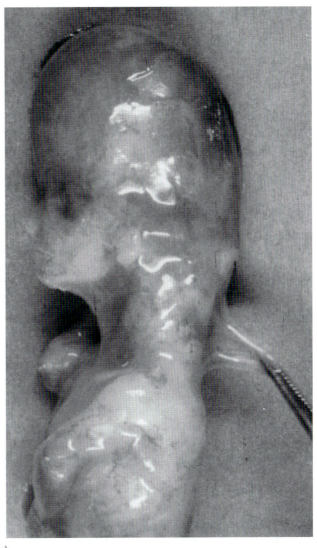

B

FIGURE 8-16 (A) Ultrasound scan at 11 weeks of gestation demonstrating 6-mm nuchal translucency (scan has been rotated 90 degrees to the left to be comparable with **B**). Chorionic villus sampling revealed trisomy 18. (*Reproduced with permission from Jackson S, Porter H, Vyas S. Ultrasound Obstet Gynecol. 1995;5:55.*) **(B)** Same fetus as shown in **A** after termination of pregnancy, demonstrating loose edematous skin over the neck, accounting for the nuchal translucency on ultrasound scanning. (*Reproduced with permission from Jackson S, Porter H, Vyas S. Ultrasound Obstet Gynecol. 1995;5:55.*)

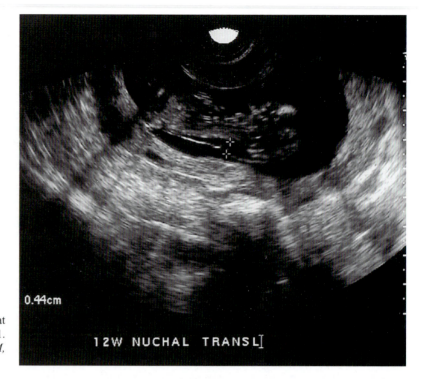

FIGURE 8-17 TVS nuchal translucency at 12 weeks of gestation in a fetus with trisomy 21. (*Reproduced with permission from Sherer DM, Manning FA. Am J Perinatol. 1999;16:103.*)

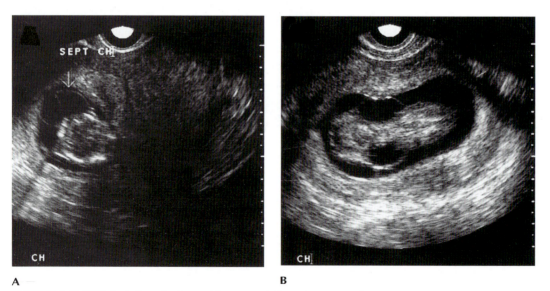

A   **B**

FIGURE 8-18 TVS depiction of a fetus with a septated first-trimester cystic hygroma. Subsequent genetic analysis demonstrated 45,X. **(A)** Transverse view of septated cystic hygroma. Note two fine, yet distinct, septations. **(B)** Coronal view of fetus. Note marked lateral projections of septated cystic hygroma. (*Reproduced with permission from Sherer DM, Manning FA. Am J Perinatol. 1999;16:103.*)

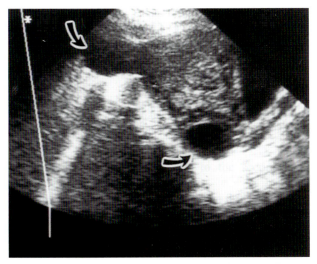

FIGURE 8-19 Complete hydatidiform mole demonstrating two theca lutein cysts (*curved arrows*), one superior to the fundus and one in the cul-de-sac.

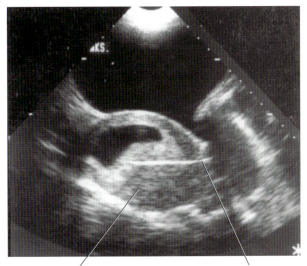

Uterine contraction   CVS catheter

FIGURE 8-20 Transcervical chorionic villus sampling catheter forced anteriorally by posterior uterine contraction.

FETAL ABDOMINAL CIRCUMFERENCE

- *See Figure 9-6.*
- Abdominal circumference is measured below heart/ above bladder and should be ovoid in shape.
- Abdominal circumference mainly reflects liver size.
- It is important in assessing intrauterine growth retardation (IUGR).
- The measurement of abdominal circumference is affected by fetal breathing, in that different shapes may be seen in inspiration/expiration.
- It is difficult to measure when there is oligohydramnios.

FETAL WEIGHT

- As determined by abdominal circumference and BPD or femur length
  - In general, ±10%
- Serial growth (percentile) is most important when IUGR is considered.
- IUGR is defined as a fetal weight in less than the 10th percentile for its age.
- The opposite, macrosomia, is a fetal weight in greater than the 90th percentile for its age, typically seen in diabetic mothers.
- There are basically two types of IUGR: asymmetric and symmetric.
  - *Asymmetric* (body smaller than head) is the most common type of IUGR. It results from or is associated with placental insufficiency—conditions that impair fetal nutrition—blood is shunted to head, glycogen stores in liver depleted.
  - *Symmetric* (both head and body too small) IUGR is usually associated with chromosomal abnormalities.
- IUGR fetuses may have learning disorders late in childhood but, most importantly, they are at risk for prenatal mortality; therefore, they need to be monitored with non-stress testing and/or biophysical profile, and umbilical artery/vein Doppler.

AMNIOTIC FLUID ASSESSMENT

- *See Figure 9-7.*
- The assessment of amniotic fluid is very subjective. The fetus should be surrounded by fluid, but not too much.
  - Too much—fetal extremity movement is unhindered.
  - Too little—fetus is crowded.
- Amniotic fluid index (AFI) is an attempt to quantify amniotic fluid volume using arbitrary vertical linear measurements in four uterine quadrants that exclude fetal body parts and the umbilical cord.
  - Less than 5 cm = oligohydramnios
  - More the 20 cm = hydramnios
- This is a very gross estimation, like saying "it is not dark until midnight."
- Amniotic fluid aspiration (amniocentesis) is performed for assessment of fetal lung maturity (lecithin: sphingomyelin ratio). It is also used for the detection of neural tube defects (elevated alpha-fetoprotein) and chromosomal abnormalities ("triple" screen—amniotic fluid alpha-fetoprotein, hCG, E_2).
- Fetal blood sampling can be accomplished by cordocentesis.

FETAL AMOMALIES

- This overview will be divided according to the organ system involved.
- For more specific information, the reader is encouraged to refer to the textbooks listed in the References section.

CENTRAL NERVOUS SYSTEM (CNS) ANOMALIES

- *See Figures 9-8 through 9-13.*
- The choroid plexus is prominent in a normal 16- to 24-week fetus.
- The atria of the lateral ventricle is normally less than 10 mm, and this stays relatively constant while the brain develops.
- The cisterna magna should be less than 10 mm.
- The mantle of the brain in a 20- to 28-week fetus can be relatively hypoechoic since it is poorly myelinated.
- Cerebellum should be dumbbell-shaped. Transcerebellar distance in mm is an estimate of the gestational age in weeks.
- Hydrocephalus refers to ventricular enlargement and subsequent head enlargement. It may be secondary to malformation or acquired as the result of an anatomic lesion.
- Common causes of hydrocephalus are:
  - Chiari type II malformation, which is associated with meningomyelocele
  - Syndromes or severe viral infection
- The basic anatomic anomaly (meningomyelocele) is associated with herniation of the brain stem structures through the foramen magnum, which in turn mechanically blocks cerebrospinal fluid flow.

- This can be recognized on sagittal images that include the cerebellum and foramen magnum. On transverse (axial) images, the cerebellum appears to be oblong in shape ("banana" sign), whereas frontal bones can also be unusually convex ("lemon" sign).
- The lateral ventricles, in particular at the atria, enlarge, and the choroid plexus shrinks.
- The atria measure over 10 mm, and the choroid plexus "dangles."
- The cisterna magna is obliterated.
- Other causes of hydrocephalus include:
  - Aqueductal stenosis, which usually occurs in males
  - Chromosomal abnormalities, which are part of syndrome
  - Holoprosencephaly: failed development of lateral ventricles may be associated with facial malformations and fused thalami
  - Masses such as teratomas of brain
  - Atrophy due to ischemia/infarct
  - Dandy-Walker malformations, which result from the obstructed foramina of Luschka and Magendie producing enlargement of the ventricle and cisterna magna

NECK AND THORACIC ANOMALIES

- *See Figures 9-14 through 9-20.*
- Cystic hygroma: malformed lymphatics at back of neck that result in septated/cystic mass
- May be associated with abdominal wall lymphangiectasia and intraperitoneal fluid seen in Turner's (XO) syndrome
- Lung mass: cystic adenomatoid malformation may be echogenic or multiple cysts
- Herniated bowel associated with diaphragmatic hernia

CARDIAC MALFORMATIONS

- *See Figures 9-21 through 9-24.*
- There is an increased risk of cardiac malformations with a history of prior pregnancy with an affected fetus, and in uncontrolled diabetes.
- In the normal heart, the right and left ventricles are about same size, and the apex of heart should tilt toward left of thorax.
- A four-chamber view should clearly document ventricles that are nearly equal in size. The interventricular septum-atrial septum may be difficult to image due to its thinness and orientation parallel to incident beam.
- Sonography should document that outflow tracts cross each other.

- Conditions associated with parallel outflow tracts include transposition of great vessels (TGV) or truncus arteriosus (TA).

RATE/RHYTHM ABNORMALITIES

- The normal fetal heart rate is between 120 and 180 beats/min.
- The rate can vary according to fetal activity and umbilical cord compression.
- Arrhythmias are common and are probably due to incompletely developed pacing centers or conduction fibers. An occasional premature contraction (either atrial or ventricular) is not uncommon.
  - Arrhythmias are usually insignificant clinically, although they may be associated with a connective tissue disorder that also attacks conduction bundles.
  - Persistent arrhythmias require a complete work-up, including fetal echocardiography.
- Signs of output failure are pericardial effusion, peritoneal fluid, and edema of soft tissue. Consider viral causes and Rh incompatibility.
- A hypoplastic left heart may have normal four chambers up to 20 weeks, then left ventricle decreases in size.
  - Can involve aorta
  - Moderator band may be mistaken as the interventricular septum

ABDOMINAL DISORDERS

- *See Figures 9-25 through 9-29.*
- Fluid should be visible within stomach of a normal fetus.
- Stomach is on left side of fetal abdomen.
- Meconium/succus entericus is seen within the bowel in a mature fetus.
- Bowel obstruction and distension can be transient.
- Diaphragmatic hernia is usually on left. Herniated bowel can displace heart and compress lungs.
- A distended stomach in duodenal atresia is associated with congenital web or Down's syndrome.
- Omphalocele versus gastroschisis:
  - *Omphalocele*: herniation of liver, sometimes bowel, through a defect at the base of the umbilical cord; has peritoneal covering. It may be associated with trisomy.
  - *Gastroschisis*: herniation of bowel through defect to right of base of umbilical cord. It is usually an isolated anomaly that may be treatable.
- Meconium peritonitis may be seen due to large bowel perforation in a fetus affected by cystic fibrosis. Echogenic collections due to calcified meconium within/on the peritoneal surfaces may be visible.

RENAL DISORDERS AND MALFORMATIONS

- *See Figures 9-30 through 9-33.*
- Normal kidneys are 3 to 5 cm in length. Mild pelvocalycectisis is normal, and is an indication of urine production.
- The collecting system should be considered distended when it is more than one-third of the anterior-posterior dimension of kidney.
- Bilateral renal agenesis is incompatible with life.
- Potter's syndrome, or severe oligohydramnios:
  - Affected fetus has low-set ears
  - Can be unilateral
- Multicystic dysplastic kidney versus ureteropelvic junction (UPJ) obstruction:
  - Ureteropelvic junction obstruction usually results in unilateral pelvocalycectesis. The cystic spaces representing distended collecting system are typically uniform in size.
  - Multicystic dysplastic kidney contains cysts of various sizes. The condition is usually unilateral, and is associated with normal amount of amniotic fluid. It occurs more often on the left and in males.
- Posterior urethral valves–bilateral fetal pelvocalycectesis
- A bladder base "keyhole" represents a distended configuration of the urethra.

SPINE ANOMALIES

- *See Figure 9-34.*
- Pedicles should line up, and be slightly flared at cervical and lumbosacral segments.
- Spine can usually be imaged adequately only in segments such as cervical, cervicothoracic, thoracolumbar, and lumbosacral.
- The spine must also be evaluated in the short axis to look for skin covering.
- Assess whether a spinal abnormality involves meningomyelocele. Try to assess level and extent of lesion (3D will be the most helpful), but fetus sometimes has back on uterine wall or placenta.
- Splaying of pedicles may indicate meningomyelocele (see earlier section on central nervous system anomalies).

LIMB ANOMALIES

- *See Figures 9-35 and 9-36.*
- Limb anomalies may be part of syndrome or separate limb resulting from amniotic band.

- The shortened long bones of dwarfism may not be apparent until the third trimester.
  - *Thanatotophoric dwarf*: shortened fermur, small thorax
  - *Achondroplastic dwarf*: shortened limbs
- Dwarfism may be associated with hydramnios.

MULTISYSTEM ANOMALIES

- *See Figure 9-37.*
- Usually part of a chromosomal syndrome, such as the Meckel-Gruber syndrome, which consists of polycystic kidney, encephalocele, and polydactyly.
- Again, the reader is encouraged to consult the textbooks listed in the References section for more detailed discussions of specific anomalies.

PLACENTAL DISORDERS

- *See Figures 9-38 through 9-42.*
- It is important to understand blood flow to, within, and from the placenta.
- The concept of trophotropism is important. The placenta can flourish (or grow or "troph") in areas of good uterine flow, and can atrophy in areas of poor uterine flow.
- The relative position of the placenta may change with uterine enlargement and the stretching of the lower uterine segment in the second trimester.
- The position of the placenta relative to internal cervical os can vary according to presence/absence of uterine contraction.
- The placenta can contain hypoechoic areas corresponding to intervillous "lakes," actual thrombosis, or subchorionic fibrin deposition. These areas typically do not have clinical importance.

ABNORMAL PLACENTAL LOCATION
- The most common placental abnormalities involve abnormal location of the placenta and placentation.
- *Placenta previa*: placenta covers area of internal cervical os.
  - Complete or central placenta previa covers the entire area of the internal cervical os.
  - Incomplete (partial) placenta previa occurs when a portion of placenta covers only limited areas around internal cervical os; also known as marginal.
  - In low-lying placenta previa, the placenta extends into the lower uterine segment.

- *Abruption placenta* can be seen as an area of hemorrhage behind the basal plate or peripherally near the marginal sinus. The area of abruption may not be visible on the scan; the area of bleeding may have decompressed by time of scanning.
- *Succenturiate lobe*: separate lobe of placenta connected to placenta proper by vessels.
- A portion of the placenta may appear as a succenturiate lobe since it is separated from the main portion of placenta, but look carefully, since one can usually connect apparent succenturiate lobe to placenta proper by scanning in all planes and by visualizing 3-dimensional placental morphology.
- *Vasa previa* is a variant of this, in which vessels cross area of internal cervical os.
- Abnormal placentation in twins: monochorionic has abnormal arterial/venous shunting (artery without accompanying vein).
- Abnormal placentation is associated with twin–twin transfusion in which one fetus is plethoric and surrounded by hydramnios, while the other is anemic and "stuck" due to the oligohydramnios and hydramnios of co-twin.

ABNORMAL PLACENTAL IMPLANTATION
- Placental implantation abnormalies involve various degrees of invasion into myometrium.
  - *Percreta*: placenta grows through myometrium into bladder wall
  - *Increta*: moderately invasive
  - *Acreta*: least invasive growth with myometrium
  - Jill Herzog's mnemonic for these: *a*creta = *a*dhered; *i*ncreta = *i*nvades; *p*ercreta = *p*erforates
  - These conditions are typically seen in C-section scars with low-lying or placenta previa.

ASSESSMENT OF PLACENTAL FUNCTION/FETAL WELL-BEING

BASIC CONCEPTS

- *See Figures 9-43 through 9-45.*
- Oxygenated blood is carried to the placenta from the uterine artery (a branch of the hypogastric internal iliac artery) to the spiral arteries. Oxygenated blood circulates into the intervillous space. Venous blood collects and returns through the marginal venous sinus. Deoxygenated blood comes back from the fetus through the placenta via the paired umbilical arteries.

They become chorionic villi arteries. Then blood empties into intervillous spaces. The venous blood circulates through the margins of cotyledon and forms the peripheral blood network of the marginal sinus.
- The placenta consists of several (10–20) cotyledons that have central arteries and peripheral venous drainage.
- Doppler interrogation of umbilical arteries reflects pressure in the intervillous space. If the pressure within intervillous space is high, it results in poor exchange. Increased intervillous pressure is reflected by decreased, absent, or reversed waveform during diastole.
- Umbilical vein flow should be phasic. If it is pulsatile, it may be an indication of high right heart pressure.
- Color Doppler sonography (CDS) can detect areas of retroplacental hemorrhage.
- Fetal intracranial flow as depicted by Doppler interrogation of the middle cerebral artery can reflect fetal condition (please see later section on fetal condition assessment).
- It can be compared to the waveform derived from the umbilical artery to reflect redistribution of flow toward the head and away from the placenta.

UMBILICAL CORD

- *See Figure 9-46.*
- The umbilical cord normally consists of one relatively large vein and two arteries.
- Lack or atrophy of artery most common, resulting in a two-vessel cord. This is associated with several fetal anomalies such as those affecting the genitourinary and gastrointestinal tracts. However, if sonography is normal and the only abnormality is the lack of a single umbilical artery, there is an approximately 7% chance of a single fetal anomaly.

FETAL CONDITION ASSESSMENT

- *See Figures 9-47 through 9-49 and Tables 9-1 and 9-2.*
- Real-time sonography can observe fetus for fetal "breathing" and body tone.
- A fetus whose condition is compromised will not exhibit "breathing"/diaphragmatic movement and will have poor body tone. This is a reflection of relative hypoxia affecting certain brain centers. Those that develop last are affected first. The first center developed is the one for fetal body tone, then heart rate variability, then breathing.

TABLE 9-1 Biophysical Profile Scoring: Technique and Interpretation

Biophysical Variable	Normal (Score = 2)	Abnormal (Score = 0)
FBM	At least one episode of FBM of at least 30 s duration in 30 min observation	Absent FBM or no episode of >30 s in 30 min
Gross body movement	At least three discrete body/limb movements in 30 min (episodes of active continuous movement considered as single movement)	Two or fewer episodes of body/limb in 30 min
Fetal tone	At least one episode of active extension with return to flexion of fetal limb(s) or trunk; opening and closing of hand considered normal tone	Either slow extension with return to partial flexion or movement of limb in full extension; absent fetal movement
Reactive FHR	At least two episodes of FHR acceleration of >15 beats/min and of at least 15 s duration associated with fetal movement in 30 min	Less than two episodes of acceleration of FHR or acceleration of <15 beats/min in 30 min
Qualitative AFV	At least one pocket of AF that measures at least 2 cm in two perpendicular planes	Either no AF pockets or a pocket <2 cm in two perpendicular planes

FBM, fetal breathing movement; FHR, fetal heart rate; AFV, amniotic fluid volume; AF, amniotic fluid.

- Changes in fetal circulation (redistribution of flow to head) can be assessed as signs of compromise in fetal condition.
- Signs of fetal blood redistribution when the fetus is hypoxic:
  - First mechanism is to shunt blood to brain. This is detected by increased diastolic flow in the middle cerebral artery waveform as compared to umbilical artery waveform (C/U ratio).
  - If this attempt to redistribute flow is insufficient, then there is increased resistance to splanchnic flow, as evidenced by increased impedance in descending abdominal aorta.
  - This also may be concomitant with increased flow through the ductus venosus.
  - Late/advanced findings are evidence of reflux in the intraheptic inferior vena cava, reversal flow in the hepatic veins associated with pulsatile flow in the umbilical vein, and absent or reversed flow in the umbilical artery Doppler waveform.
- The most severely compromised fetus has absent/reversed diastolic flow in the umbilical artery.
- Uteroplacental flow can be assessed by Doppler interrogation of the uterine artery as it branches off the hypogastric (internal iliac) artery.
- A diastolic notch is normal up to approximately 26 weeks. If present, it may indicate a potential to develop toxemia of pregnancy-induced hypertension (PIH).
- This is related to a lack of trophoblastic invasion of the spiral arteries and failure to transformed coiled vessels to become open-mouthed (large capacity) sinuses.

TABLE 9-2 Interpretation of Fetal Biophysical Profile Score Results and Recommended Clinical Management

Test Score Result	Interpretation	PNM Within 1 wk Without Intervention	Management
10 of 10 8 of 10 (normal fluid), 8 of 8 (NST not done)	Risk of fetal asphyxia extremely rare	1 per 1000	Intervention only for obstetric and maternal factors; no indication for intervention for fetal disease
8 of 10 (abnormal fluid)	Probable chronic fetal compromise	89 per 1000	Determine that there is functioning renal tissue and intact membranes; if so, deliver for fetal indications
6 of 10 (normal fluid)	Equivocal test, possible fetal asphyxia	Variable	If the fetus is mature, deliver; in the immature fetus, repeat test within 24 h; if <6/10, deliver
6 of 10 (abnormal fluid)	Probable fetal asphyxia	89 per 1000	Deliver for fetal indications
4 of 10	High probability of fetal asphyxia	91 per 1000	Deliver for fetal indications
2 of 10	Fetal asphyxia almost certain	125 per 1000	Deliver for fetal indications
0 of 10	Fetal asphyxia certain	600 per 1000	Deliver for fetal indications

PNM, perinatal mortality; NST, nonstress test.

CERVICAL INCOMPETENCE

- *See Figures 9-50 through 9-52.*
- Transvaginal sonography (TVS) provides detailed assessment of cervical length and configuration.
- The cervix can also be imaged using a transperineal approach.
- A normal cervix is at least 2.5 cm in length (from internal cervical os to external os), with no bulging or funneling.
- When there is incompetence, the cervix at the internal cervical os has a V configuration, which progresses to a U.

DELIVERY DECISIONS

- Timing of delivery is determined by assessment of fetal age, well-being, and weight.
- Mode: vaginal versus "operative" (C-section).
- Large masses such as fibroids in the lower uterine segment may preclude vaginal bleeding.
- Place: at a general hospital versus at tertiary care center with level III neonatal intensive care, if needed.

KEY FUNDAMENTAL CONCEPTS

- Sonography has a vital role in the assessment of fetal development and well-being in mid- and late pregnancy.
- It also provides for assessment of the placenta, including its location, morphology, and physiology.
- Fetal structural defects can be detected by sonography, including those affecting the central nervous, cardiovascular, gastrointestinal, genitourinary, and musculoskeletal systems.
- Multiple anomalies may indicate certain syndromes.
- Sonographic assessment of fetal condition can be accomplished with a biophysical profile and Doppler parameters.

REFERENCES

Benacerraf B. *Ultrasound of Fetal Syndromes.* New York: Churchill-Livingstone, 1998.

Benson CB, Doubilet PM. The fetal genitourinary system. In: Fleischer AC, Manning F, Jeanty P, Romero R, eds. *Sonography in Obstetrics and Gynecology: Principles and Practice*, ed. 6. New York: McGraw-Hill, 2001:431.

Emerson DS. Color Doppler sonography in obstetrics. In: Fleischer AC, Manning F, Jeanty P, Romero R, eds. *Sonography in Obstetrics and Gynecology: Principles and Practice*, ed. 6. New York: McGraw-Hill, 2001:315.

Fleischer AC. Sonography of the umbilical cord and intrauterine membranes. In: Fleischer AC, Manning F, Jeanty P, Romero R, eds. *Sonography in Obstetrics and Gynecology: Principles and Practice*, ed. 6. New York: McGraw-Hill, 2001:225.

Gervasi M-T, Romero R, Maymon E, Pacora P, Jeanty P. Ultrasound examination of the uterine cervix during pregnancy. In: Fleischer AC, Manning F, Jeanty P, Romero R, eds. *Sonography in Obstetrics and Gynecology: Principles and Practice*, ed. 6. New York: McGraw-Hill, 2001:821.

Ghezzi F, Romero R, Maymon E, Redman M, Blackwell S, Berry SM. Fetal blood sampling. In: Fleischer AC, Manning F, Jeanty P, Romero R, eds. *Sonography in Obstetrics and Gynecology: Principles and Practice*, ed. 6. New York: McGraw-Hill, 2001:775.

Goncalves LF, Romero R, Gervasi M-T, Maymon E, Pacora P, Pilu G. Doppler velocimetry of the uteroplacental circulation. In: Fleischer AC, Manning F, Jeanty P, Romero R, eds. *Sonography in Obstetrics and Gynecology: Principles and Practice*, ed. 6. New York: McGraw-Hill, 2001:285.

Goncalves LF, Romero R, Maymon E, Pacora P, Bianco K, Jeanty P. Prenatal detection of anatomic congenital anomalies. In: Fleischer AC, Manning F, Jeanty P, Romero R, eds. *Sonography in Obstetrics and Gynecology: Principles and Practice*, ed. 6. New York: McGraw-Hill, 2001:141.

Harman C. Ultrasound in the management of the alloimmunized pregnancy. In: Fleischer AC, Manning F, Jeanty P, Romero R, eds. *Sonography in Obstetrics and Gynecology: Principles and Practice*, ed. 6. New York: McGraw-Hill, 2001:683.

Hertzburg BS, Kliewer MA, Bowie JD. Sonography of the fetal gastrointestinal system. In: Fleischer AC, Manning F, Jeanty P, Romero R, eds. *Sonography in Obstetrics and Gynecology: Principles and Practice*, ed. 6. New York: McGraw-Hill, 2001:409.

Jeanty P. Fetal biometry. In: Fleischer AC, Manning F, Jeanty P, Romero R, eds. *Sonography in Obstetrics and Gynecology: Principles and Practice*, ed. 6. New York: McGraw-Hill, 2001:139.

Jeanty P, Clavelli WA, Romaris SS. Ultrasound detection of chromosomal anomalies. In: Fleischer AC, Manning F, Jeanty P, Romero R, eds. *Sonography in Obstetrics and Gynecology: Principles and Practice*, ed. 6. New York: McGraw-Hill, 2001:583.

Jeanty P, Goncalves LF. Neck and chest fetal anomalies. In: Fleischer AC, Manning F, Jeanty P, Romero R, eds. *Sonography in Obstetrics and Gynecology: Principles and Practice*, ed. 6. New York: McGraw-Hill, 2001:389.

Joern H, Funk A, Coetz M, Kuehlwein H, Klein A, Fendel H. Development of quantitative Doppler indices for uteroplacental and fetal blood flow during the third trimester. *Ultrasound Med Biol.* 1996;22:823.

Manning FA. Fetal biophysical profile score: theoretical consideration and practical application. In: Fleischer AC, Manning F, Jeanty P, Romero R, eds. *Sonography in Obstetrics and Gynecology: Principles and Practice*, ed. 6. New York: McGraw-Hill, 2001:711.

Manning FA. Ultrasound-guided fetal invasive therapy: current status. In: Fleischer AC, Manning F, Jeanty P, Romero R, eds. *Sonography in Obstetrics and Gynecology: Principles and Practice*, ed. 6. New York: McGraw-Hill, 2001:805.

Manning FA. Intrauterine growth restriction: diagnosis, prognostication, and management based on ultrasound methods. In: Fleischer AC, Manning F, Jeanty P, Romero R, eds. *Sonography in Obstetrics and Gynecology: Principles and Practice*. New York: McGraw-Hill, 2001:615.

Mari G, Detti L. Doppler ultrasound: application of fetal medicine. In: Fleischer AC, Manning F, Jeanty P, Romero R, eds. *Sonography in Obstetrics and Gynecology: Principles and Practice*, ed. 6. New York: McGraw-Hill, 2001:247.

Maymon E, Romero R, Ghezzi F, Pacora P, Pilu G, Jeanty P. Fetal skeletal anomalies. In: Fleischer AC, Manning F, Jeanty P, Romero R, eds. *Sonography in Obstetrics and Gynecology: Principles and Practice*, ed. 6. New York: McGraw-Hill, 2001:445.

Maymon E, Romero R, Goncalves L, Gervasi M-T, Redman M, Ghezzi F. Amniocentesis. In: Fleischer AC, Manning F, Jeanty P, Romero R, eds. *Sonography in Obstetrics and Gynecology: Principles and Practice*, ed. 6. New York: McGraw-Hill, 2001:741.

Pilu G, Jeanty P, Perolo A, Prandstraller D. Prenatal diagnosis of congenital heart disease. In: Fleischer AC, Manning F, Jeanty P, Romero R, eds. *Sonography in Obstetrics and Gynecology: Principles and Practice*, ed. 6. New York: McGraw-Hill, 2001:157.

Pilu G, Romero R, Gabrielli S, Perolo A, Bovicelli L. Prenatal diagnosis of cerebrospinal anomalies. In: Fleischer AC, Manning F, Jeanty P, Romero R, eds. *Sonography in Obstetrics and Gynecology: Principles and Practice*, ed. 6. New York: McGraw-Hill, 2001:375.

Reyes J, Concalves LF, Silva SR, Jeanty P. Sonography of multiple gestations. In: Fleischer AC, Manning F, Jeanty P, Romero R, eds. *Sonography in Obstetrics and Gynecology: Principles and Practice*, ed. 6. New York: McGraw-Hill, 2001:637.

Rizzo G, Capponi A, Romanini C. Fetal functional echocardiography. In: Fleischer AC, Manning F, Jeanty P, Romero R, eds. *Sonography in Obstetrics and Gynecology: Principles and Practice*, ed. 6. New York: McGraw-Hill, 2001:177.

Silva SR, Jeanty P. Fetal syndromes. In: Fleischer AC, Manning F, Jeanty P, Romero R, eds. *Sonography in Obstetrics and Gynecology: Principles and Practice*, ed. 6. New York: McGraw-Hill, 2001:507.

Spirt BA, Gordon LP. Sonography of the placenta. In: Fleischer AC, Manning F, Jeanty P, Romero R, eds. *Sonography in Obstetrics and Gynecology: Principles and Practice*, ed. 6. New York: McGraw-Hill, 2001:195.

Wapner RJ. Chorionic villus sampling. In: Fleischer AC, Manning F, Jeanty P, Romero R, eds. *Sonography in Obstetrics and Gynecology: Principles and Practice*, ed. 6. New York: McGraw-Hill, 2001:721.

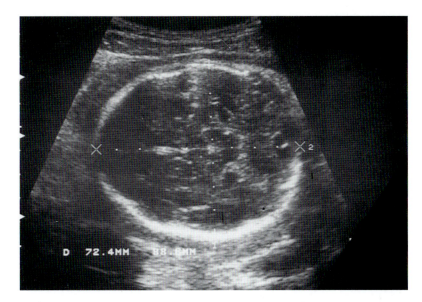

FIGURE 9-1 Biparietal diameter is measured at the level of the thalamus from the outer to the inner skull.

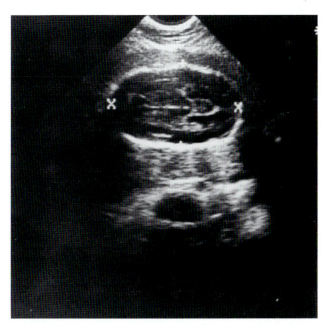

FIGURE 9-2 Example of dolichocephaly in a fetus that has premature rupture of the membrane.

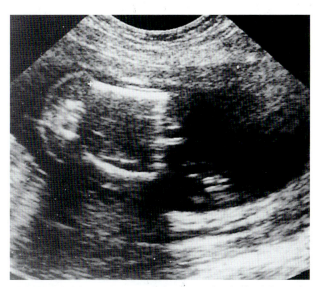

FIGURE 9-3 Measurement of the femur is obtained from the most proximal portion of the shaft to the distal end. Neither the femoral head nor the distal epiphysis is included. When two femurs are seen in the same section, only the proximal one is measured. Acoustical shadowing from one femur or from other bones can artifactually decrease the length of the other femur.

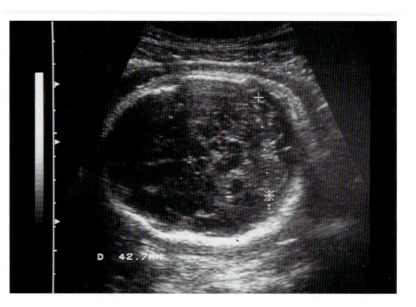

FIGURE 9-4 Cerebrellar measurement is taken as the longest widths of the cerebrellar hemispheres.

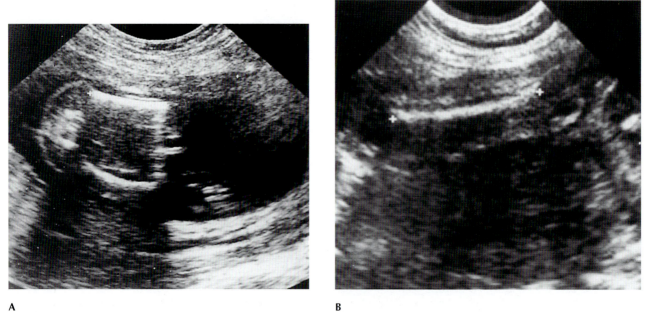

A

B

FIGURE 9-5 (A) Measurement of the femur is obtained from the most proximal portion of the shaft to the distal end. Neither the femoral head nor the distal epiphysis is included. When two femurs are seen in the same section, only the proximal one is measured. Acoustical shadowing from one femur or from other bones can artifactually decrease the length of the other femur. **(B)** Measurement of the humerus is obtained in the same way as measurement of the femur.

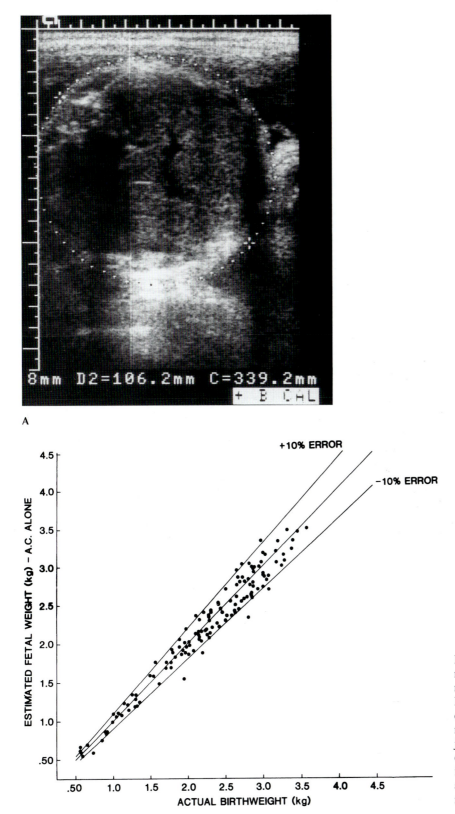

8mm D2=106.2mm C=339.2mm

+ B CHL

A

B

FIGURE 9-6 Ultrasound estimation of fetal mass. **(A)** Abdominal circumference is measured at the level of the fetal liver. Because the upper fetal abdomen is cylindrical in shape, there is little variation in measured circumference if the liver and major hepatic veins are present. **(B)** Abdominal circumference (AC) gives an estimate of fetal weight to within a 15% error in nearly all instances and to within ±10% in the majority of instances. *(Figure continued.)*

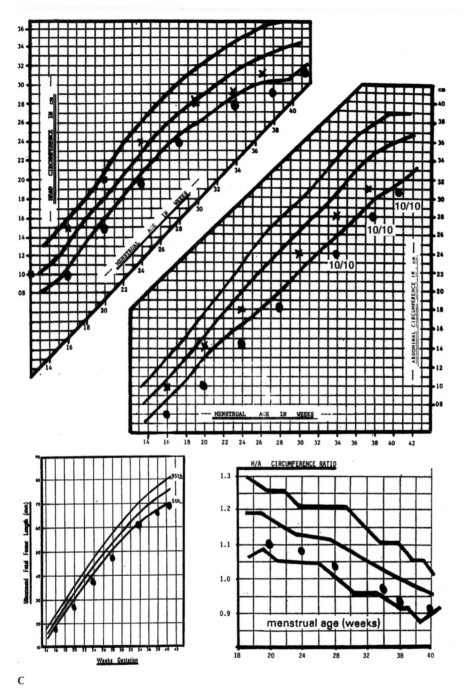

C

FIGURE 9-6 *(continued)* The role of serial fetal morphometrics and functional assessment of well-being in the diagnosis and management of intrauterine growth restriction (IUGR). **(C)** One fetus presents with a discrepancy of 4 weeks between fetal age by menstrual history (•) and, at initial ultrasound, morphometrics (*). Fetal growth velocity, intrafetal proportions, and functional parameters are consistently normal. H/A, head/abdomen.*(Figure continued.)*

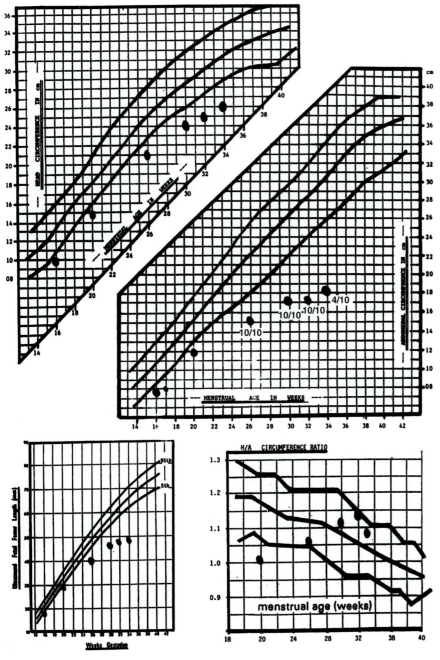

D

FIGURE 9-6 *(continued)* **(D)** The second fetus with uncertain menstrual dates demonstrates late onset (26 weeks), diminished growth velocity, and progressive change in intrafetal proportions, and at 34 weeks developed evidence of functional compromise (biophysical profile score 4/10, oligohydramnios).

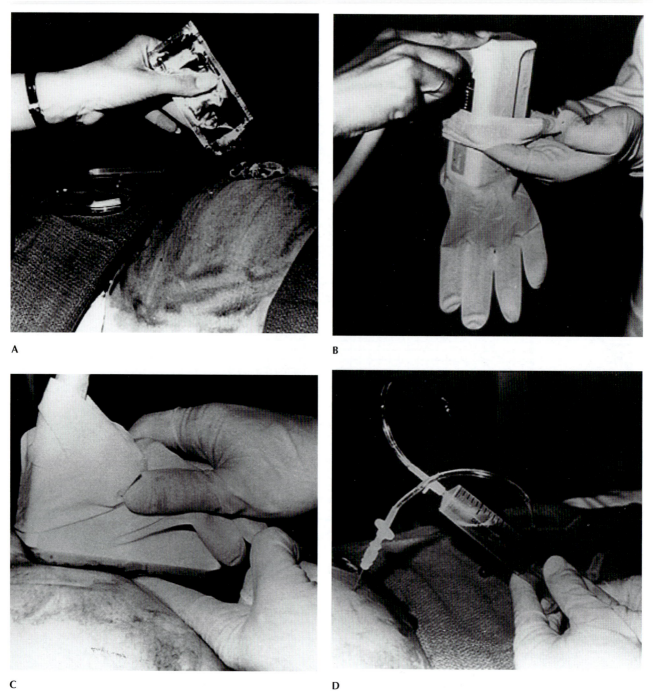

A

B

C   D

FIGURE 9-7 (A) Preparation of a sterile field using antiseptic and sterile drapes and application of sterile gel. **(B)** Insertion of the transducer into a sterile glove. **(C)** Placing the gloved finger at the puncture site, underneath the linear transducer, produces a shadow in the ultrasound image that allows identification of the needle path. **(D)** Withdrawal of amniotic fluid using a 22-gauge needle, extension tubing, and a 20-cc syringe.

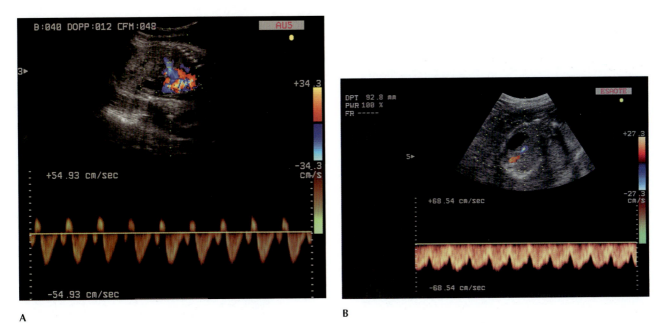

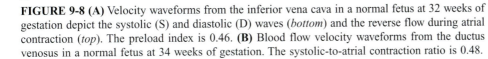

FIGURE 9-8 (A) Velocity waveforms from the inferior vena cava in a normal fetus at 32 weeks of gestation depict the systolic (S) and diastolic (D) waves (*bottom*) and the reverse flow during atrial contraction (*top*). The preload index is 0.46. **(B)** Blood flow velocity waveforms from the ductus venosus in a normal fetus at 34 weeks of gestation. The systolic-to-atrial contraction ratio is 0.48.

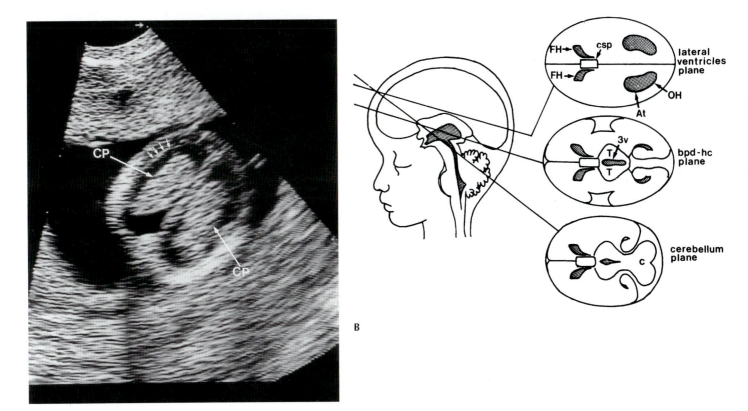

FIGURE 9-9 (A) Transvaginal sonogram (TVS). At 12 weeks' gestation, the brightly echogenic choroid plexuses (CP) dominate the intracranial cavity. The thin sonolucent cortex is also demonstrated (*arrows*). **(B)** Three scanning planes that allow visualization of the relevant intracranial fetal anatomy. From rostrad to caudad, the first plane demonstrates the lateral ventricles; the second plane is used to measure biparietal diameter (bpd) and head circumference (hc); the third plane reveals the cerebellum within the posterior fossa. FH, frontal horns; csp, cavitas septi pellucidum; At, atrium; OH, occipital horn; T, thalami; 3v, third ventricle; c, cerebellum.

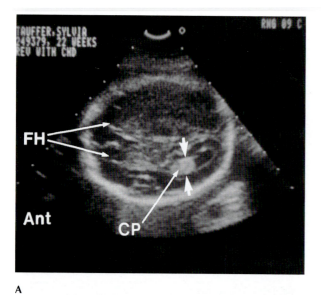

A

B

FIGURE 9-10 Axial scans at similar levels in a normal fetus and in a fetus with hydrocephalus. **(A)** Normalcy is indicated by the brightly echogenic choroid plexus (CP) that entirely fills the lumen of the atrium, being closely opposed to both medial and lateral walls of the ventricle (*arrowheads*). **(B)** Hydrocephalus is indicated by the anterior displacement of the shrunken choroid plexus, which appears clearly detached from the medial wall of the ventricle. FH, frontal horns of lateral ventricles; Ant, anterior; Post, posterior.

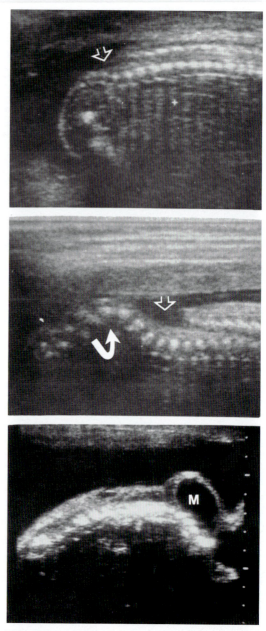

FIGURE 9-11 Sagittal views demonstrating spectrum of spina bifida. From top to bottom, sacral spina bifida (*open arrow*), thoracolumbar spina bifida (*open arrow*) with severe associated kyphoscoliosis, and complete rachischisis with cervical meningocele (M). (*Reproduced with permission from Pilu G, Romero R, Reece EA, et al. Am J Obstet Gynecol. 1988;158:1052.*)

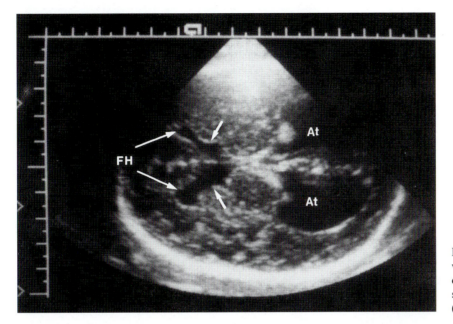

FIGURE 9-12 Hydrocephalus in a fetus with spina bifida. Hypertrophy of the caudate nucleus (*arrows*) results in a typical square appearance of the frontal horns (FH). At, atria of lateral ventricles.

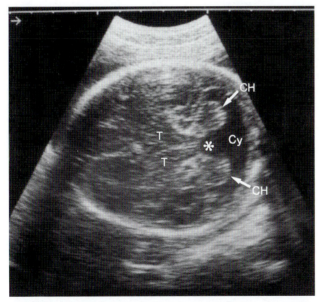

FIGURE 9-13 The fourth ventricle (*) amply communicates with a cystic cisterna magna (Cy) through a wide defect of the cerebellar vermis. Cerebellar hemispheres (CH) are widely separated. This is Dandy-Walker malformation. T, thalami.

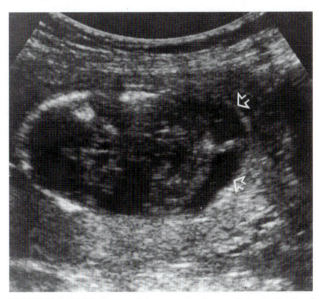

FIGURE 9-14 Fluid-containing masses (*arrows*) in the back of the neck of a fetus, with a septation in the middle. These are characteristic of the mild form of cystic hygroma.

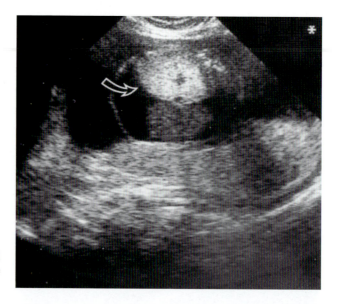

FIGURE 9-15 This echogenic mass (*arrow*) associated with pleural effusion represents type III cystic adenomatoid malformation of the lung.

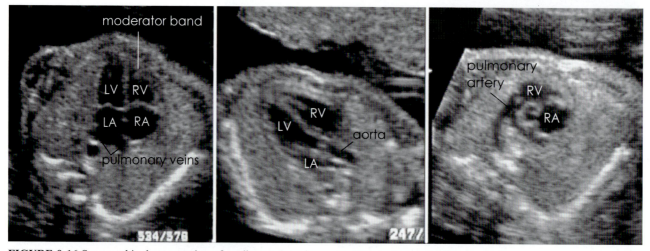

FIGURE 9-16 Sonographic demonstration of cardiac anatomy in a normal second-trimester fetus: four-chamber view (*left*), left heart view (*middle*), and right heart view (*right*). LA and LV, left atrium and ventricle, respectively; RA and RV, right atrium and ventricle, respectively.

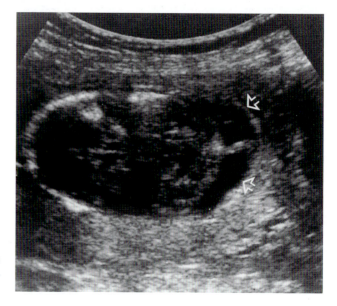

FIGURE 9-17 Fluid-containing masses (*arrows*) in the back of the neck of a fetus, with a septation in the middle. These are characteristic of the mild form of cystic hygroma.

218

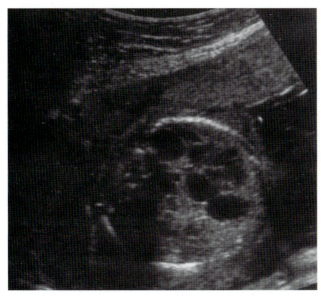

A

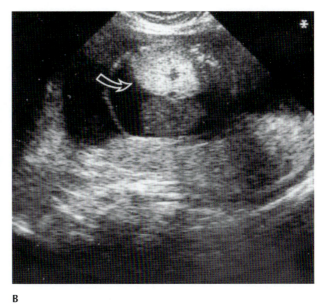

B

FIGURE 9-18 (A) Numerous cysts in the chest that represent type I cystic adenomatoid malformation. Some of the cysts were drained under ultrasound guidance but reappeared within 48 h. **(B)** This echogenic mass (*arrow*) associated with pleural effusion represents type III cystic adenomatoid malformation of the lung.

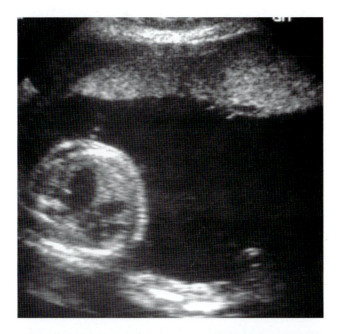

FIGURE 9-19 Typical appearance of diaphragmatic hernia, with the stomach alongside the heart, the shift of the heart, and polyhydramnios.

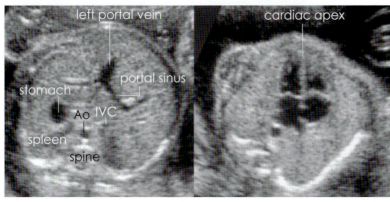

FIGURE 9-20 Sonographic assessment of the visceral situs. In a transverse scan of the abdomen, the stomach, spleen, and abdominal aorta are seen on the left; the portal sinus, gallbladder (*not shown*), and inferior vena cava are seen on the right. In a transverse section of the chest, the cardiac apex is seen pointing to the left.

219

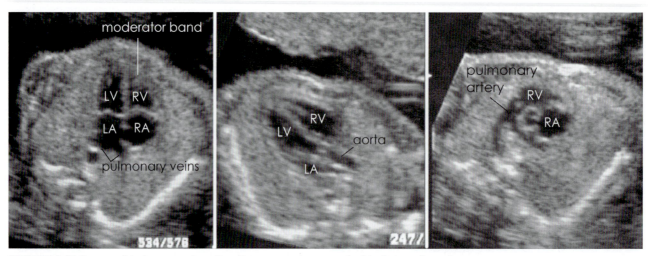

FIGURE 9-21 Sonographic demonstration of cardiac anatomy in a normal mid-trimester fetus: four-chamber view (*left*), left heart view (*middle*), and right heart view (*right*). LA and LV, left atrium and ventricle, respectively; RA and RV, right atrium and ventricle, respectively.

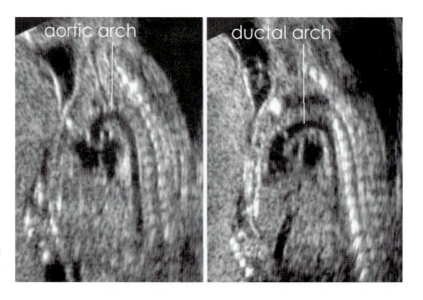

FIGURE 9-22 Aortic and ductal arches. The long upward course and the presence of the brachiocephalic vessels identify the aortic arch.

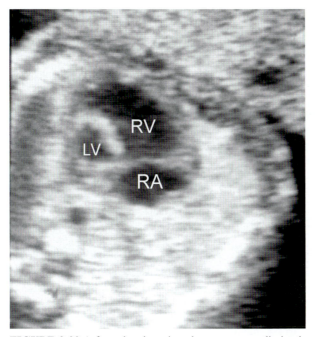

FIGURE 9-23 A four-chamber view demonstrates a diminutive left ventricle (LV) with a bright and thickened endocardium and no contractility in real-time examination, indicating hypoplastic left heart syndrome.

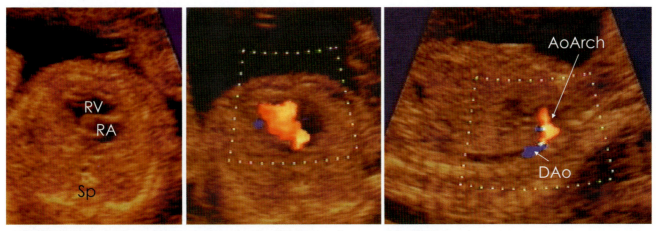

FIGURE 9-24 The left heart chambers are not visualized. Color Doppler sonography (CDS) demonstrates only one patent atrioventricular valve and reversed flow within the aortic arch (AoArch), indicating hypoplastic left heart syndrome. Sp, spine; DAo, descending aorta.

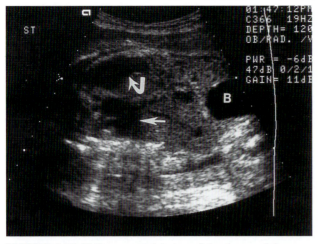

FIGURE 9-25 Oblique coronal image of the thorax, abdomen, and pelvis of a fetus with a diaphragmatic hernia. The stomach (*curved arrow*) is not seen in its expected location in the left upper quadrant but is instead seen in the thorax, adjacent to the heart (*straight arrow*). B, bladder.

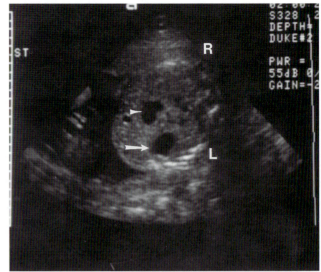

FIGURE 9-26 Axial image of a fetus with duodenal atresia shows a "double bubble" sign due to fluid in the stomach (*arrow*) in the left upper quadrant and a dilated duodenal bulb (*arrowhead*) on the right. L, toward fetal left; R, toward fetal right.

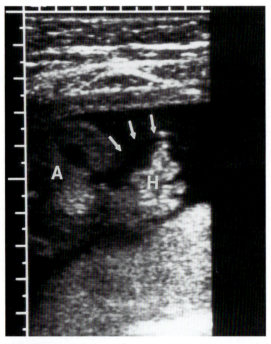

FIGURE 9-27 Fetus with gastroschisis. Note normal insertion of umbilical cord (*arrows*) into the fetal abdomen (A). H, herniated bowel.

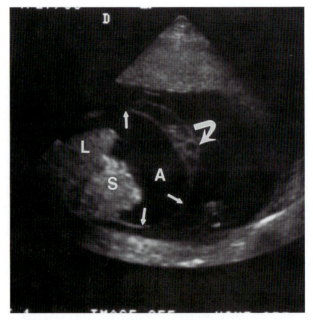

FIGURE 9-28 Scan through the eviscerated contents of an omphalocele shows both the liver (L) and the small bowel (S) surrounded by ascites (A) and a membrane (*straight arrows*). Note the insertion of the umbilical cord (*curved arrow*) onto the membrane surrounding the omphalocele.

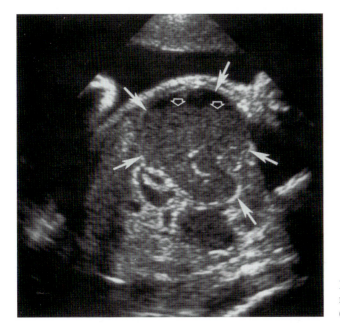

FIGURE 9-29 Oblique image through the abdomen of a fetus with meconium peritonitis demonstrating a large meconium pseudocyst (*solid arrows*) with a fluid debris level (*open arrows*).

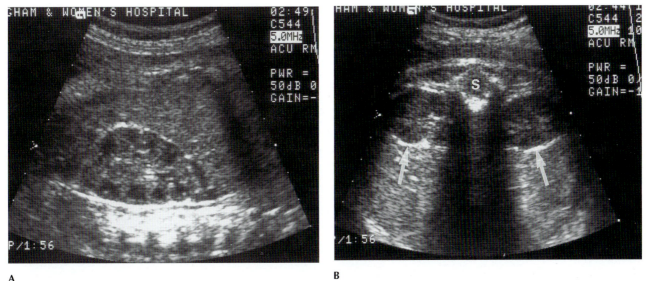

A

B

FIGURE 9-30 Normal kidneys. **(A)** Longitudinal scan of a normal kidney demonstrating its reniform shape with central sinus echoes and hypoechoic pyramids. **(B)** Transverse view of both kidneys (*arrows*), one on either side of the spine (S), which casts a shadow between them.

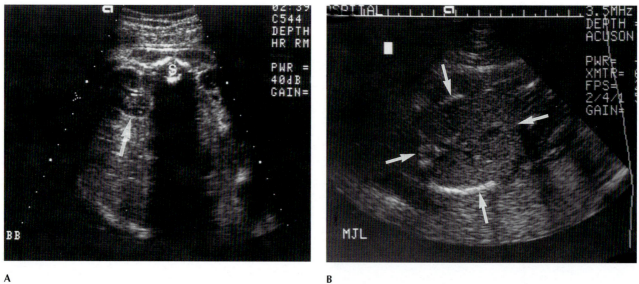

A   B

FIGURE 9-31 (A) Unilateral renal agenesis. Transverse view at the level of the kidneys demonstrating one kidney (*arrow*) to the right of the spine (S) and no kidney on the left. **(B)** Bilateral renal agenesis. Transverse view of the fetal abdomen (*arrows*) demonstrating severe oligohydramnios and no kidneys.

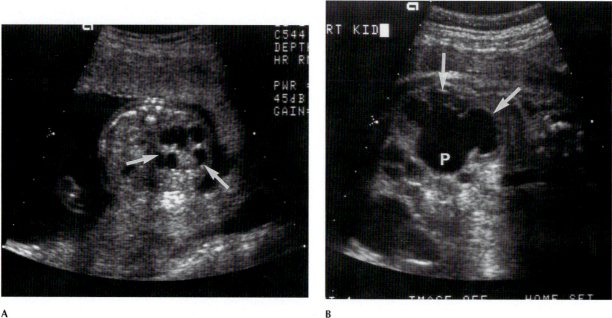

A   B

FIGURE 9-32 (A) Multicystic dysplastic kidney. Transverse sonogram of fetal abdomen demonstrating dysplastic kidney as a cluster of cysts with a small amount of solid tissue (*arrows*) in the renal fossa. **(B)** Hydronephrosis. Coronal view of a hydronephrotic kidney showing a dilated renal pelvis (P) and dilated calyces (*arrows*). *(Figure continued.)*

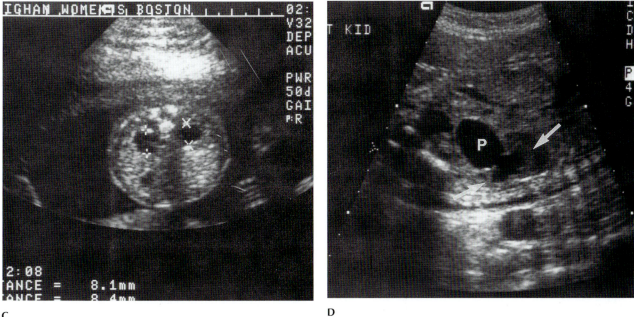

C

D

FIGURE 9-32 *(continued)* **(C)** Transverse view of hydronephrotic kidneys with dilated renal pelvises measured anterior to posterior (*calipers*). **(D)** Ureteropelvic junction obstruction. Coronal view of kidney (*arrows*) obstructed at the ureteropelvic junction with a markedly dilated renal pelvis (P) and dilated intrarenal collecting system.

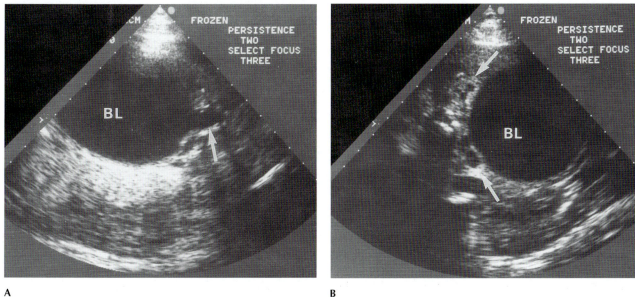

A

B

FIGURE 9-33 Posterior urethral valves. **(A)** Longitudinal view of pelvis showing enlarged bladder (BL) with dilated posterior urethra (*arrow*). **(B)** Transverse view of fetal abdomen showing markedly dilated bladder (BL) and small, echogenic, dysplastic kidneys (*arrows*).

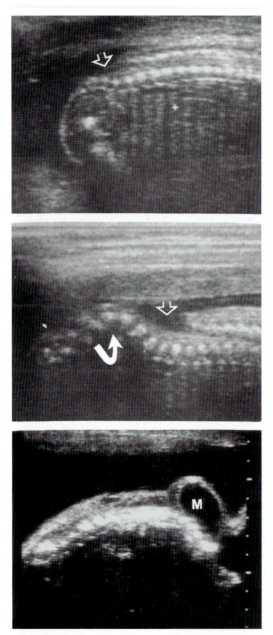

FIGURE 9-34 Sagittal views demonstrating spectrum of spina bifida. From *top* to *bottom*, sacral spina bifida (*open arrow*), thoracolumbar spina bifida (*open arrow*) with severe associated kyphoscoliosis, and complete rachischisis with cervical meningocele (M). (*Reproduced with permission from Pilu G, Romero R, Reece EA, et al. Am J Obstet Gynecol. 1988;158:1052.*)

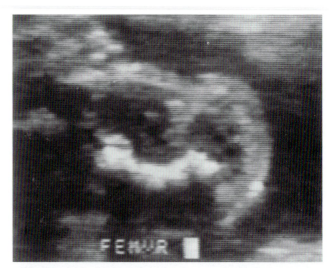

FIGURE 9-35 Bowed and short femur with the typical "telephone receiver" appearance.

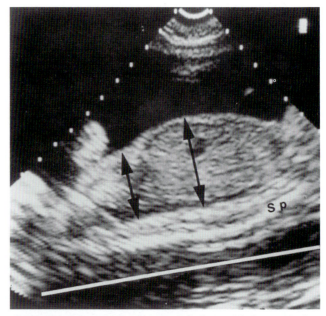

FIGURE 9-36 Longitudinal section of a fetus with thanatophoric dysplasia. Note the significant disproportion between the chest and abdomen. Sp, spine. (*Reproduced with permission from Jeanty P, Romero R. Obstetrical Ultrasound. New York: McGraw-Hill, 1983.*)

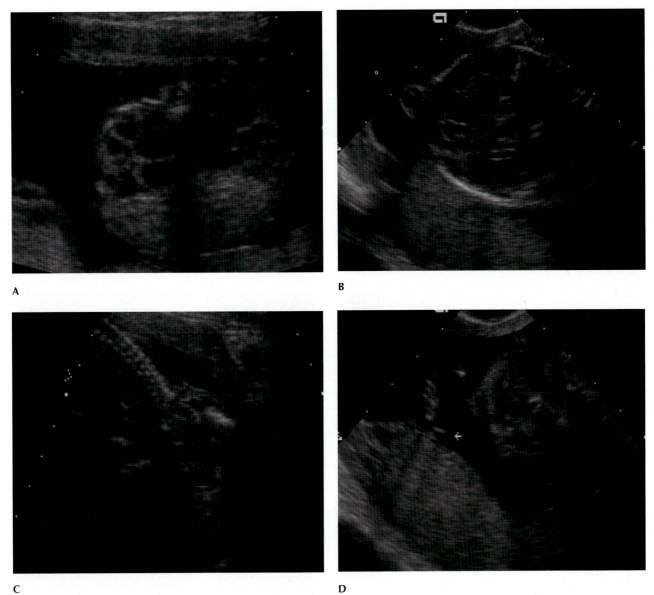

A

B

C

D

FIGURE 9-37 (A) Large bilateral cystic kidneys that resemble multicystic kidneys. The amniotic fluid is normal, which is atypical. **(B)** An 8-mm posterior cephalocele in axial **(B)** and sagittal **(C)** views. **(D)** Postaxial polydactyly (arrow).

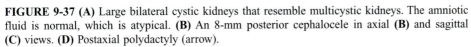

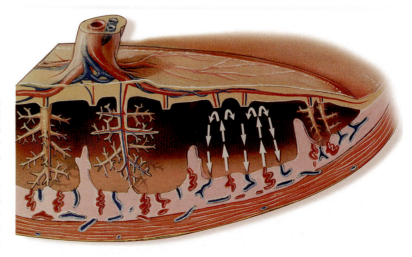

FIGURE 9-38 Blood flow to, within, and from placenta. Oxygenated blood arrives from the spiral artery and bathes the intervillous space. Excess blood traverses the peripherally located venous sinuses. From the intervillous space, blood travels to the fetus through the chorionic villous veins. Numerous chorionic villous vessels fuse to become the umbilical vein, which carries oxygenated blood to fetus. Deoxygenated blood returns from the fetus via the paired umbilical arteries, which bathe the chorionic villi vessels within the placenta.

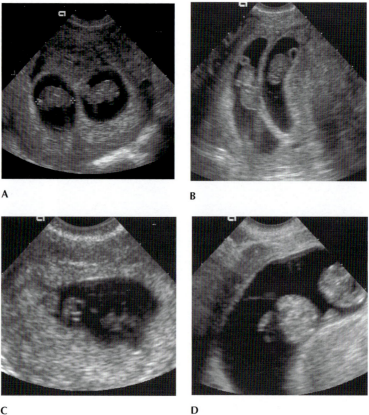

FIGURE 9-39 The two top images show dichorionic twins, which are easily recognized from the monochorionic twins on the two bottom images (first trimester) by the thick intervening membrane.

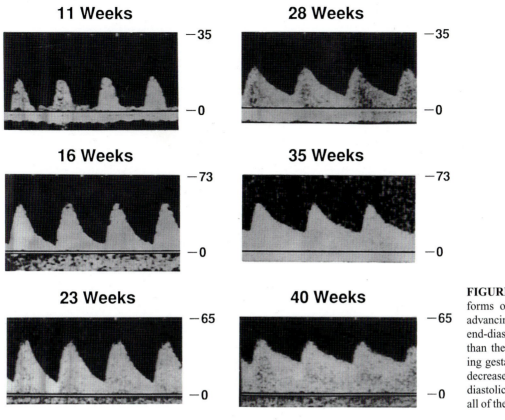

11 Weeks

−35

−0

28 Weeks

−35

−0

16 Weeks

−73

−0

35 Weeks

−73

−0

23 Weeks

−65

−0

40 Weeks

−65

−0

FIGURE 9-40 Flow velocity waveforms of the umbilical artery with advancing gestation. Note that the end-diastolic velocity increases more than the peak velocity with advancing gestation. This is quantified by a decreased pulsatility index, systolic/diastolic ratio, or resistance index, or all of these, with advancing gestation.

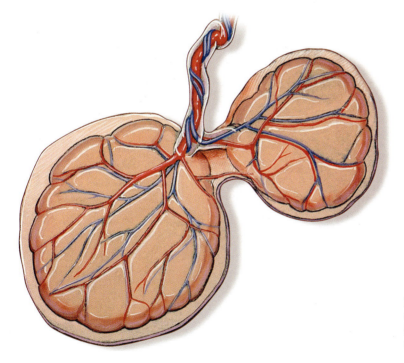

FIGURE 9-41 The succenturiate lobe can contain vessels that have little support. If these vessels cross the internal cervical os they are potentially the cause of excessive bleeding (vasa previa).

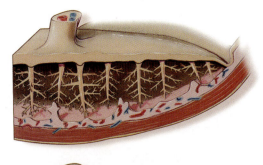
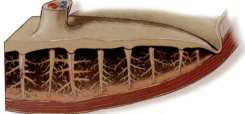
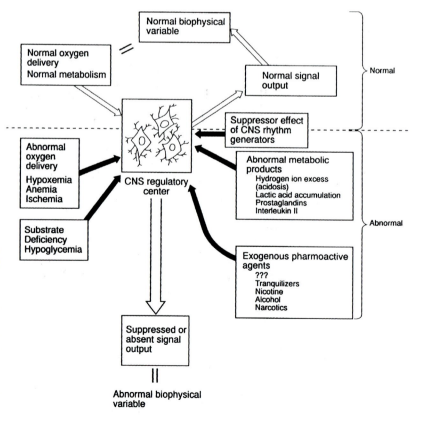

FIGURE 9-42 Various degrees of vascular invasion of the myometrium. (*Top*) Normal basal plate with spiral arteries and veins separate from the underlying myometrium. (*Middle*) Vascular invasion into deep myometrium (acreta). (*Bottom*) Vascular invasion past myometrium into surrounding tissues (increta, percreta).

FIGURE 9-43 A schematic of the factors, both normal and pathologic and both intrinsic and extrinsic, that modulate dynamic fetal biophysical activities. The observation of a normal given biophysical activity is strong presumptive evidence that the central nervous system (CNS) regulatory neurons are not hypoxic. In contrast, the failure to observe a variable necessitates a differential diagnosis. (*Reproduced with permission from Manning FA, ed. Fetal Medicine: Principles and Practice. Norwalk, CT: Appleton & Lange, 1995.*)

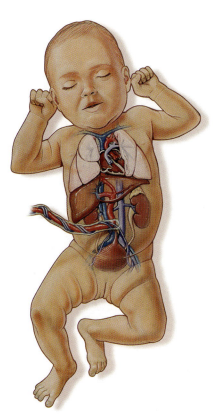

FIGURE 9-44 Fetal circulation. Oxygenated blood is carried toward the fetus in the umbilical vein. The umbilical vein then carries blood into the liver via the ductus venosus, which directly courses into the inferior vena cava, or through the middle hepatic vein. Blood may also pass into the portal sinus within the liver. Blood then courses to the right atrium where it can travel across the foramen ovale into the left atrium or down into the right ventricle. Then blood moves into the ductus arteriosus and into the aorta, where it is directed either toward the head or into the splanchnic circulation. Blood returning through the pulmonary veins courses through the left atrium and left ventricle into the aorta. Deoxygenated blood returns to the placenta via the paired umbilical arteries.

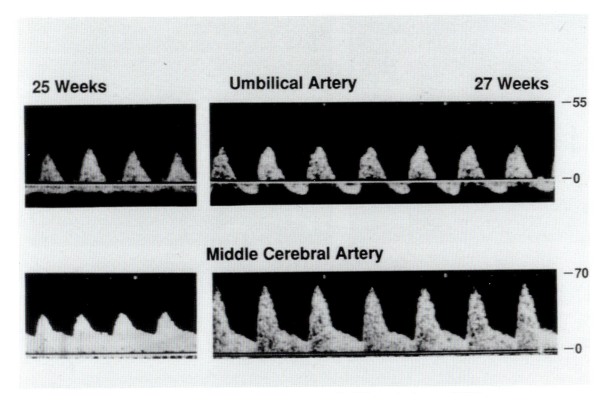

FIGURE 9-45 Flow velocity waveforms of the umbilical artery and middle cerebral artery (MCA) at 25 and 27 weeks of gestation in a severely growth-retarded fetus. At 25 weeks there was absent end-diastolic velocity of the umbilical artery flow velocity waveforms (FVW), pulsation of the umbilical vein, and the brain-sparing effect (shown by high diastole of the MCA). At 27 weeks there was reverse-diastolic FVW of the umbilical artery, and the brain-sparing effect was not present. The fetus died 24 h after this study. (*Reproduced with permission from Mari G, Wasserstrum N.* Am J Obstet Gynecol. *1991;164:776.*)

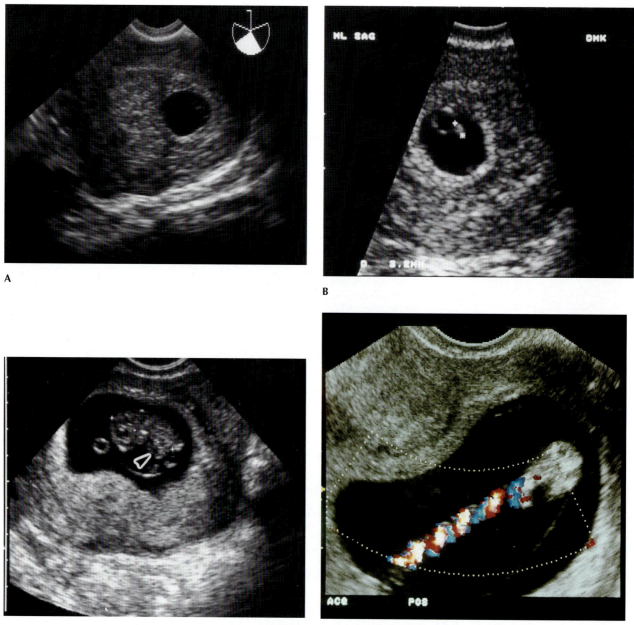

FIGURE 9-46 Development of the umbilical cord. **(A)** TVS at 5 weeks shows "double bleb" corresponding to the amnion and yolk sac on either side of the embryo. **(B)** Same as **A,** 5 days later. The yolk sac/embryo complex is depicted clearly. The embryo measures 3 mm in length. **(C)** Developing umbilical cord at 8 weeks. There is a suggestion of bowel herniating into the base of the cord *(arrowhead)*. The yolk sac is extraamniotic. **(D)** CDS shows the umbilical cord at 10 weeks. *(Figure continued.)*

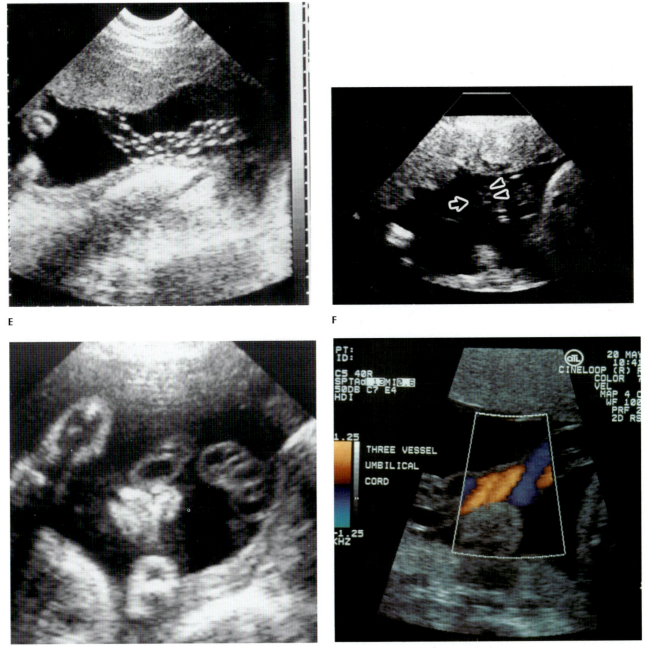

E

F

G

H

FIGURE 9-46 *(continued)* **(E)** Long axis of the umbilical cord in a 20-week pregnancy demonstrates the spiral course of umbilical arteries. **(F)** Sonographic image of normal umbilical cord depicted in true short axis shows two arteries (*arrowheads*) adjacent to the single umbilical vein (*large arrow*). **(G)** Normal umbilical cord adjacent to the fetal face demonstrates the vein and two arteries in oblique section. **(H)** Normal umbilical cord has two arteries (in red) coiling around the central single vein as depicted with amplitude CDS. *(Figure continued.)*

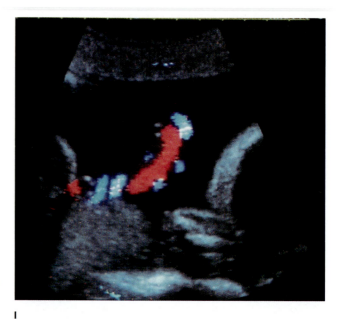

FIGURE 9-46 *(continued)* **(I)** CDS of normal umbilical cord, with vein depicted as red and arteries depicted as blue.

I

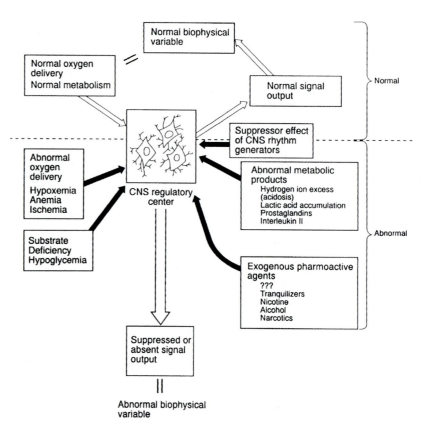

FIGURE 9-47 A schematic of the factors, both normal and pathologic and both intrinsic and extrinsic, that modulate dynamic fetal biophysical activities. The observation of a normal given biophysical activity is strong presumptive evidence that the central nervous system (CNS) regulatory neurons are not hypoxic. In contrast, the failure to observe a variable necessitates a differential diagnosis. (*Reproduced with permission from Manning FA, ed. Fetal Medicine: Principles and Practice. Norwalk, CT: Appleton & Lange, 1995.*)

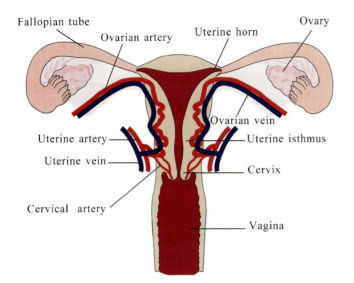

A

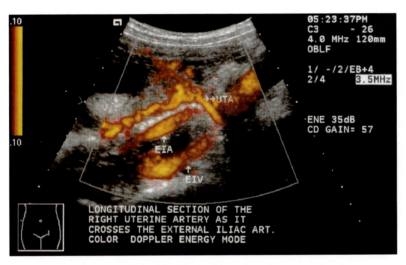

B

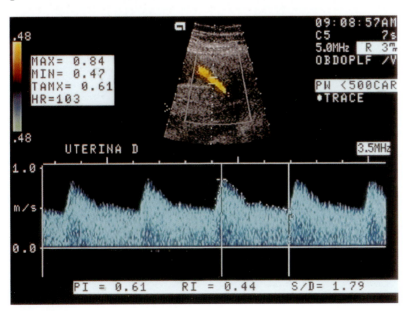

C

FIGURE 9-48 (A) Blood supply to the uterus. (*Reproduced with permission from Cunningham FG, MacDonald PC, Gant NF, et al. In: Cunningham FG, MacDonald PC, Leveno K, Gilstrap LC II, eds.* Williams Obstetrics. *Norwalk, CT: Appleton & Lange, 1993:57.*) **(B)** Color Doppler energy picture showing the uterine artery at its apparent cross with the external iliac artery. This is the preferred site to obtain a waveform. **(C)** Normal uterine artery velocity waveform. Note the high velocities during diastole.

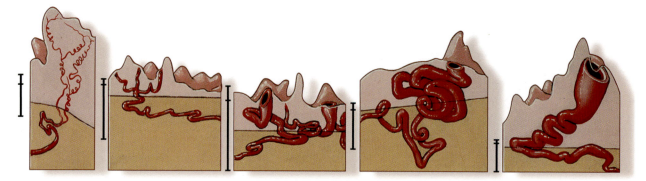

FIGURE 9-49 Transformation of spiral arteries throughout pregnancy. They start as thin, coiled vessels. Then there is gradual enlargement of the vessel openings due to trophoblastic infiltration of the muscular media of the vessel. They eventually form open-mouthed vessels that afford high capacitance. If this process is incomplete, pregnancy-induced hypertension (PIH) may occur resulting in poor flow to the fetus. The bars at the left of the images depict the relative thickness of the endometrium and myometrium. The drawings depict the spiral arteries at approximately 6-8 weeks, 12-14 weeks, 20-22 weeks, 26-28 weeks, and 32-34 weeks.

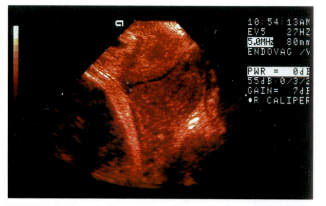

FIGURE 9-50 TVS of a normal uterine cervix; the internal os, the external os, and the endocervical canal can be easily visualized.

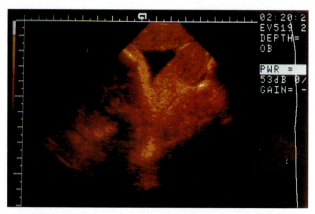

FIGURE 9-51 TVS of a cervix with a V-shaped funnel.

FIGURE 9-52 Distribution of cervical length at 23 weeks of gestation in 2702 low-risk patients. (*Reproduced with permission from Health VCF, et al. Ultrasound Obstet Gynecol. 1998;12:312.*)

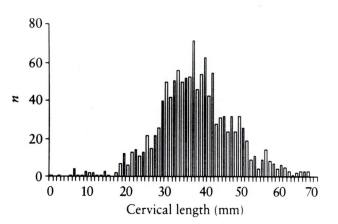

10 MATERNAL DISORDERS

OVERVIEW

- Sonography is used for assessment of the pregnant woman in a variety of ways, including assessment of pelvo/abdominal pain associated with appendicitis, renal calculi, pelvic masses, and fibroids, and for evaluation of breast masses.

APPENDICITIS

- *See Figure 10-1.*
- The appendix is usually displaced cephalically by a gravid uterus.
- An inflamed appendix appears as a noncompressible fusiform structure adjacent to the right side of uterus. The appendiceal walls are thickened (greater than 6 mm). Sometimes only the mesentery is inflamed.

RENAL CALCULI

- The renal pelvis becomes distended after 16 to 18 weeks of pregnancy.
- The distension may be secondary to increased renal volume flow and/or relaxation of pelvocalyceal tone.
- Calculi tend to lodge within the ureter at the ureteropelvic junction, at the level of the pelvic brim, or at the ureterovesicular junction.

PELVIC MASSES

- *See Figures 10-2 and 10-3.*
- Corpus luteum of pregnancy is a normal structure until 14 to 16 weeks.
- In the case of a cystic septated mass, consider cystadenoma.
- A fibroid, which is a common solid mass arising or adjacent to uterus, can enlarge during pregnancy, driven by high estrogen levels. A fibroid can also undergo accelerated degeneration infarction, causing pain.
- Adnexal torsion may also cause pain during pregnancy.
- Adnexal torsion may produce enlarged ovaries with little or no intraovarian venous flow. (Please refer to Chapter 6 for a more detailed discussion.)

BREAST MASSES

- *See Figures 10-4 through 10-11.*
- A breast mass may enlarge during pregnancy.
- Sonography can be particularly useful in pregnant patients since typically breasts are very dense on mammography during pregnancy.
- Sonography has an important role in distinguishing cysts from solid masses such as fibroadenoma.
- A solid mass with an irregular border suggests malignancy, especially if it has a spiculated border, which indicates tumor infiltration into surrounding soft tissue.

KEY FUNDAMENTAL CONCEPTS

- Sonography is useful in evaluating mothers who experience pelvic pain during pregnancy. It can be used for identification of renal calculi, diagnosis of appendicitis, or evaluation of a pelvic mass, with or without torsion.
- Sonography is also accurate in distinguishing breast cysts from other solid masses.

REFERENCES

Cosgrove D. Breast ultrasound. In: Fleischer AC, Manning F, Jeanty P, Romero R, eds. *Sonography in Obstetrics and Gynecology: Principles and Practice*, ed. 6. New York: McGraw-Hill, 2001:1207.

Fleischer AC, Wheeler TC. Sonography of maternal disorders. In: Fleischer AC, Manning F, Jeanty P, Romero R, eds. *Sonography in Obstetrics and Gynecology: Principles and Practice*, ed. 6 New York: McGraw-Hill, 2001:869.

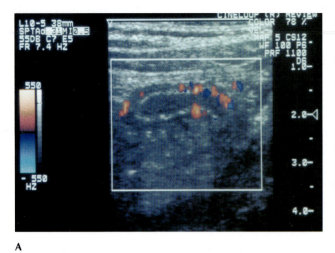

A

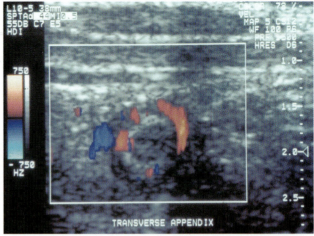

B

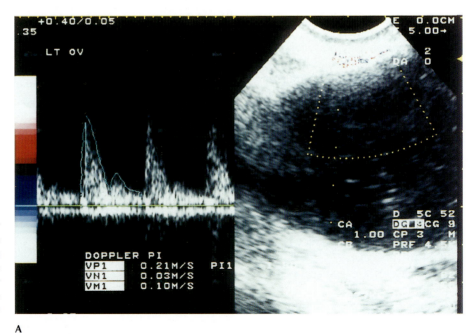

C

FIGURE 10-1 Appendicitis. **(A, B)** Transabdominal color Doppler sonogram (CDS) of appendicitis showing thickened and hyperemic appendiceal wall in long **(A)** and short **(B)** axes. (*Courtesy of ATL, Inc.*) **(C)** Thickened appendiceal wall (*between cursors*) in a patient with right lower quadrant pain. An unruptured appendix with acute inflammation was found at surgery.

FIGURE 10-2 Transvaginal color Doppler sonogram (TV-CDS) of benign and malignant ovarian masses in pregnant patients. **(A)** Mostly cystic mass with high-impedance flow within the wall. This was a cystadenoma at surgery. *(Figure continued.)*

A

238

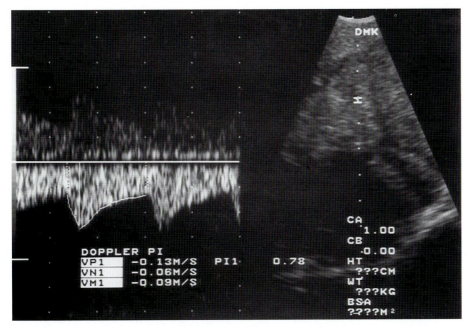

B

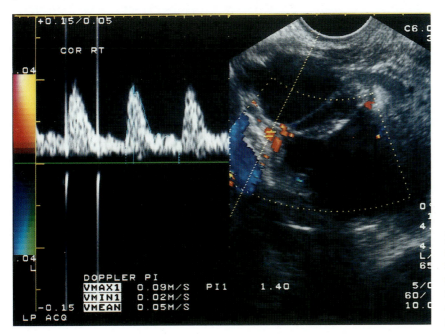

C

FIGURE 10-2 *(continued)* **(B)** Complex predominantly solid mass with low-impedance flow found at cesarean section to represent an ovarian carcinoma. **(C)** TV-CDS showing high-impedance flow within a mucinous cystadenoma appearing as a septated, mostly cystic mass. *(Figure continued.)*

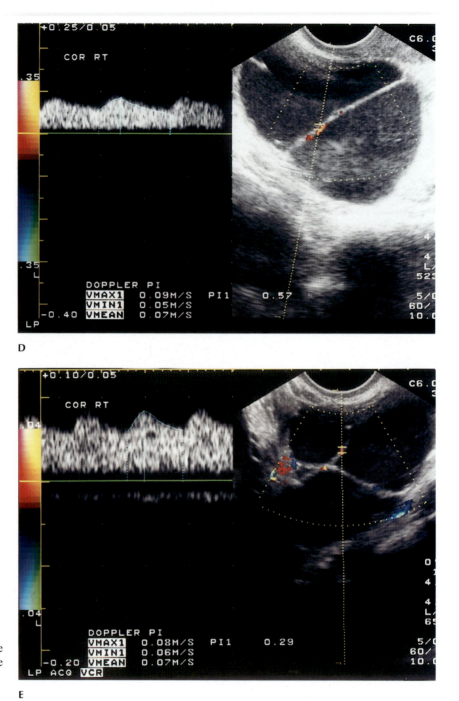

FIGURE 10-2 *(continued)* **(D, E)** Same patient as in **C,** showing low-impedance flow with the mucinous cystadenoma.

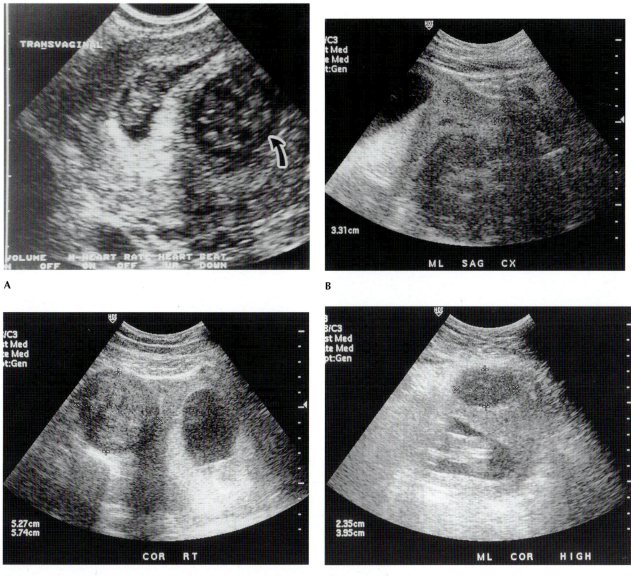

FIGURE 10-3 (A) Transvaginal sonogram (TVS) of 8-week intrauterine pregnancy, showing a fibroid (*curved arrow*) in the lower uterine segment. The fibroid is a stationary, well-defined area of hypoechogenicity, as opposed to a uterine contraction, which blends into surrounding myometrium. **(B, C, D)** Multiple fibroids in a 16-week intrauterine pregnancy. **(B)** A large (6 × 8 cm) fibroid displaces the cervix (*between cursors*). **(C)** There is a subserosal fundal fibroid (*between cursors*). **(D)** A smaller fibroid (*between cursors*) is also seen as a well-circumscribed hypoechoic area within the anterior wall of the uterus. *(Figure continued.)*

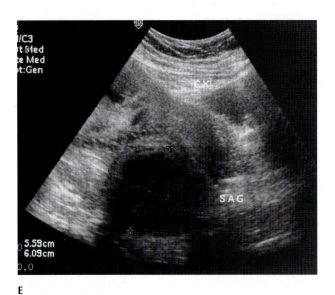

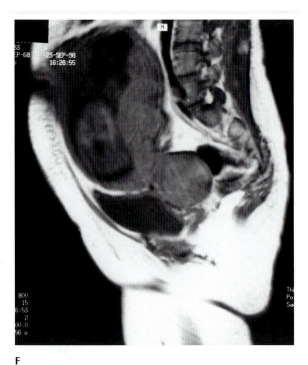

E   F

FIGURE 10-3 *(continued)* **(E)** A large fibroid (*between cursors*) displaces the cervix anteriorly. Its exact location and origin could not be ascertained with TVS. **(F)** Magnetic resonance imaging (T$_1$-weighted, midline sagittal) shows the fibroid to be pedunculated, probably arising from the posterior aspect of the lower uterine segment.

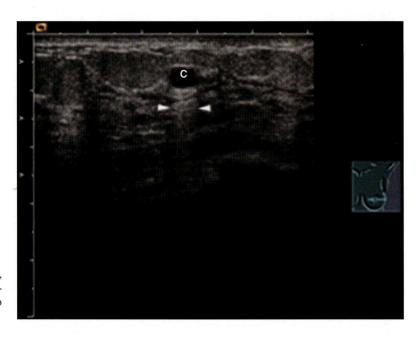

FIGURE 10-4 Breast cyst. This well-defined, echo-free lesion with increased sound transmission (*arrowheads*) is typical of a simple cyst. No further investigation is needed. C, cyst.

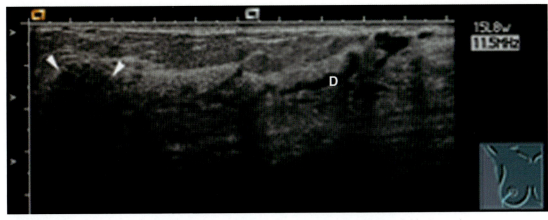

FIGURE 10-5 Fibroadenoma. The well-defined margins and regular oval shape of this 5-mm lesion (*calipers*) are typical features of a fibroadenoma, as is the uniform low level of echoes. It also lies horizontally in the breast and shows increased sound transmission (*arrows*). D, duct.

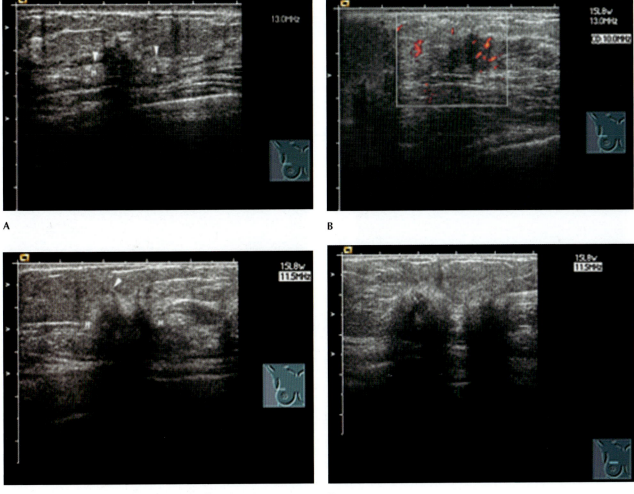

FIGURE 10-6 Breast carcinomas. **(A)** The subcentimeter carcinoma shows the typical features, with a poorly defined echogenic halo surrounding the echo-poor nidus, which casts an acoustic shadow. **(B)** The tissue planes are broken (*arrowheads*) and on the power Doppler study the lesion is markedly vascular. **(C)** A larger tumor also shows these features, and there is thickening of the Cooper's ligaments (*arrowheads*), producing a stellate pattern converging on the lesion and drawing attention to it. **(D)** Multicentric cancers are not uncommon and should be carefully sought.

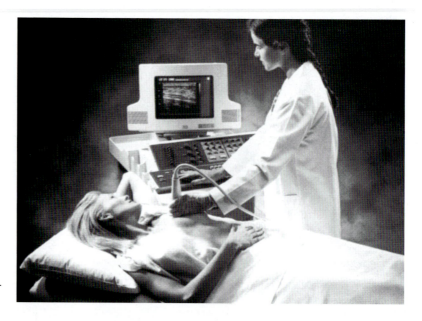

FIGURE 10-7 A breast sonogram being performed with a Philips/ATL 5000.

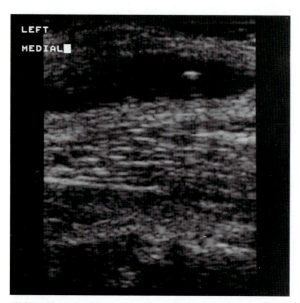

FIGURE 10-8 Oblong-shaped breast cyst during needle aspiration. The tip of the needle is echogenic.

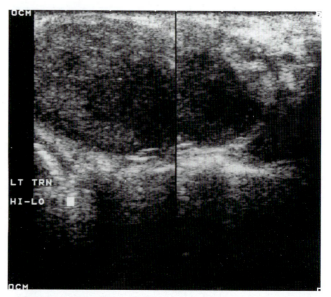

FIGURE 10-9 Composite image of well-circumscribed solid breast mass representing a fibroadenoma.

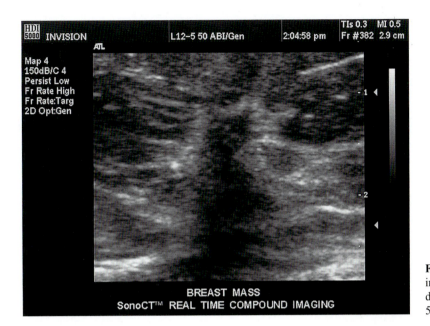

FIGURE 10-10 Magnified SonoCT image showing an irregular solid mass with speculated borders, an indication of tumor invasion. This was a 5-mm breast cancer.

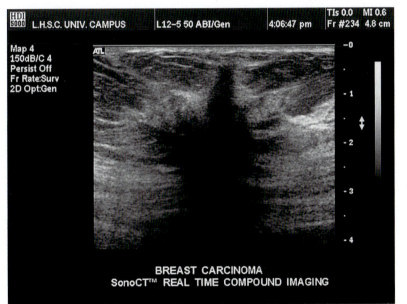

FIGURE 10-11 SonoCT image of 4-mm breast cancer detected by its shadowing due to surrounding tissue invasion and fibrosis.

11 NEW AND FUTURE DEVELOPMENTS

OVERVIEW

- Sonography is an exciting discipline. New developments are happening all the time, primarily due to improved signal processing.
- Sonography can provide a means to better understand disease processes and their response to treatment.

3D AND 4D

- *See Figures 11-1 through 11-3.*
- 3D sonography is commercially available now on most mid-to-high-range scanners.
- 3D affords images not obtainable with 2D.
- Must be user-friendly, easy to use, and quick.
- Surface rendition best for depiction of fetal face, limbs, and meningomyelocele.
- Minimum ("see through") intensity plot used for assessment of cardiac structures.
- Volume mode obtains data for evaluation in different selectable scan planes.
- The operator should interact with the 3D data set to optimize the diagnostic value of 3D.
- 4D is 3D displayed in real time, also referred to as live-3D.

CONTRAST ENHANCEMENT

- *See Figures 11-4 through 11-6.*
- Best agent is a 3-micron microbubble.
- Provides for assessment of blood flow and relative vascularity.
- Contrast can determine "wash-in" and "wash-out" enhancement kinetics.
- Contrast affords enhanced depiction of tumor vascularity.
- Improved depiction of vascularity with contrast may afford detection of tumor or areas of ischemia and/or necrosis.

- Contrast enhancement may also be helpful for assessment of tubal patency and anatomy.

KEY FUNDAMENTAL CONCEPTS

- Recent improvements in image processing have allowed for the development of 3D and 4D sonography, which in turn should improve assessment of normal and abnormal anatomy.
- Use of contrast will allow assessment of blood flow, which could provide an objective means to monitor physiologic processes.
- Sonography is a versatile and user-friendly modality that will continue to improve its ability to provide anatomic and physiologic parameters.

REFERENCES

Downey DB, Fenster A, Williams J. Clinical utility of three-dimensional US. *R.S.N.A.* 1995;20:559.

Fleischer AC, Donnelly EF. Three-dimensional color power sonography in gynecology: (C) Three-dimensional color Doppler sonography of fibroids preembolization and postembolization. In: Fleischer AC, Manning F, Jeanty P, Romero R, eds. *Sonography in Obstetrics and Gynecology: Principles and Practice*, ed. 6. New York: McGraw-Hill, 2001:1245.

Kurjak A, Kupesic S. Three-dimensional color power sonography in gynecology: (A) Three-dimensional power Doppler in the assessment of pelvic tumor angiogenesis. In: Fleischer AC, Manning F, Jeanty P, Romero R, eds. *Sonography in Obstetrics and Gynecology: Principles and Practice*, ed. 6. New York: McGraw-Hill, 2001:1225.

Lee W, Chaiworapongsa T, Romero R, et al. A diagnostic approach for the evaluation of spina bifida by three-dimensional ultrasonography. *J. Ultrasound Med.* 2002;21:619.

Orden M-R, Gudmundsson S, Kirkinen P. Contrast-enhanced sonography in the examination of benign and malignant adnexal masses. *J. Ultrasound Med.* 2000;19:783.

Pairleitner H. Three-dimensional color power sonography in gynecology: (B) Three-dimensional color Doppler sonography histogram: a new way of quantify blood flow. In: Fleischer AC, Manning F, Jeanty P, Romero R, eds. *Sonography in Obstetrics and Gynecology: Principles and Practice*, ed. 6. New York: McGraw-Hill, 2001:1241.

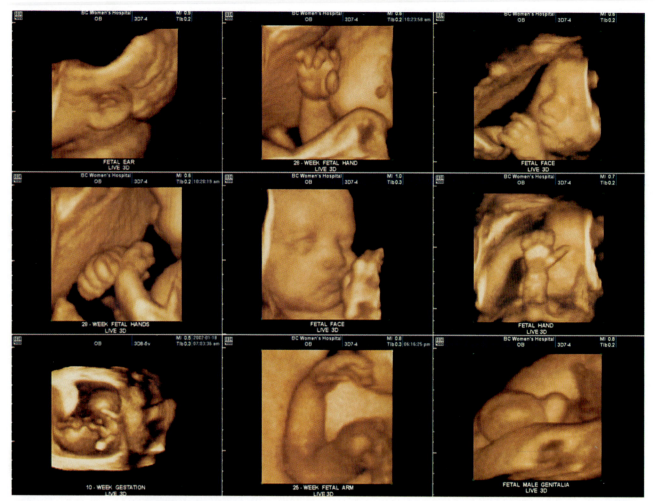

FIGURE 11-1 Composite of 3D sonograms of a variety of fetal anatomy. (*Courtesy of Philips/ATL, Inc.*)

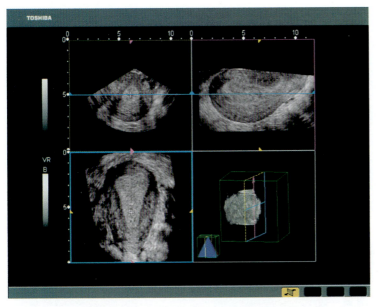

A

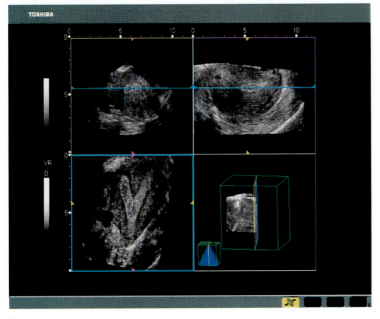

B

FIGURE 11-2 3D sonography of the uterus. (*Courtesy of Toshiba America Medical Systems, Inc.*) **(A)** A composite of short and long axis of a normal uterus (*top images*) with reconstructed coronal (*bottom left*) and volume rendering (*bottom right*). **(B)** As compared to **A**, there is a V configuration of the endometrium with a smooth fundal contour diagnostic of a septated uterus.

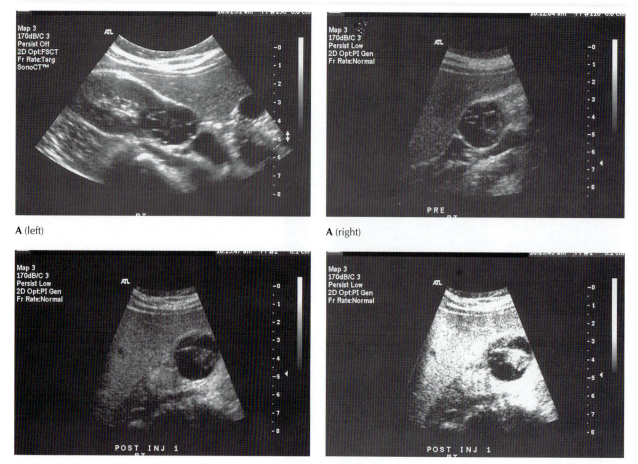

A (left)

A (right)

B (left)

B (right)

FIGURE 11-3 Contrast-enhanced sonography. **(A)** Initial transabdominal sonogram of septated cystic renal mass in long (*left*) and short (*right*) axes. **(B)** With contrast, the septated areas and solid portions of the mass are enhanced. (*Left*) Low mechanical index (MI) and (*right*) high MI images. This was a papillary renal cancer.

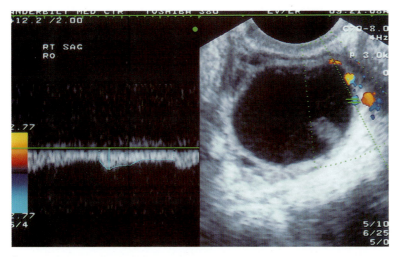

A

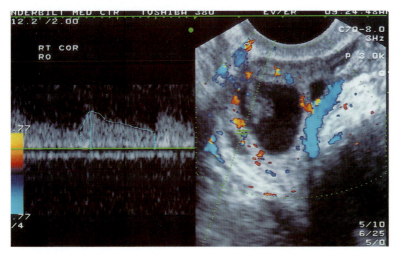

B

FIGURE 11-4 Flow within solid area of benign versus malignant cystic tumors. **(A, B)** No flow was detected within solid area in this corpus luteum cyst, which regressed between the initial scan **(A)** and the follow-up scan 6 weeks later **(B)**. Low-impedance flow is present in the solid area within an ovarian cancer.

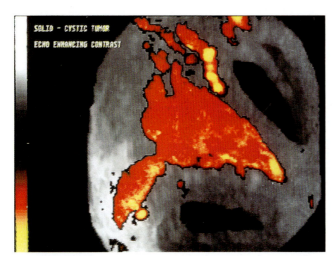

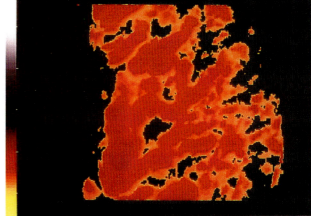

FIGURE 11-5 The same patient as in Figure 11-4, 2 min after application of contrast medium. Note tortuous vessels with irregular branching, indicative of ovarian malignancy. This was confirmed by histopathology.

FIGURE 11-6 Three-dimensional power Doppler scan of ovarian carcinoma neoangiogenesis enhanced by injection of the contrast agent. Numerous randomly dispersed vessels with irregular branching are obtained in minute intervals (1 to 3 min) to observe possible differences in the filling and wash-out phase.

Appendix 1
American College of Radiology (ACR) Standard for the Performance of an Ultrasound Examination of the Female Pelvis

I. INTRODUCTION

- This standard has been developed to provide assistance to physicians performing ultrasound studies of the female pelvis. Ultrasound of the female pelvis should be performed only when there is a valid medical reason, and the lowest possible ultrasonic exposure settings should be used to gain the necessary diagnostic information. In some cases, additional or specialized examinations may be necessary. While it is not possible to detect every abnormality, adherence to the following standard will maximize the probability of detecting most of the abnormalities that occur.

II. QUALIFICATIONS OF PERSONNEL

- See the ACR Standard for Performing and Interpreting Diagnostic Ultrasound Examinations.

III. SPECIFICATIONS OF THE ULTRASOUND EXAMINATION OF THE FEMALE PELVIS

- The following standard describes the examination to be performed for each organ and anatomic region in the female pelvis. All relevant structures should be identified by the transabdominal or transvaginal approach. In many cases, both will be needed.

A. GENERAL PELVIC PREPARATION

- For a pelvic sonogram performed transabdominally, the patient's urinary bladder should be adequately distended. For a transvaginal sonogram, the urinary bladder is usually empty. The vaginal transducer may be introduced by the patient, the sonographer, or the sonologist. It is recommended that a woman be present in the examining room during a transvaginal sonogram, either as an examiner or a chaperone.

B. UTERUS

- The vagina and uterus provide anatomic landmarks that can be utilized as reference points for the remaining normal and abnormal pelvic structures. In evaluating the uterus, the following should be documented: a) the uterine size, shape, and orientation; b) the endometrium; c) the myometrium; and d) the cervix. The vagina may be imaged as a landmark for the cervix and lower uterine segment.
- Uterine size can be obtained. Uterine length is evaluated in long axis from the fundus to the cervix (the external os, if it can be identified). The depth of the uterus (anteroposterior dimension) is measured in the same long-axis view from its anterior to posterior walls, perpendicular to the length. The width is measured from the transaxial or coronal view.
- Abnormalities of the uterus should be documented. The endometrium should be analyzed for thickness, echogenicity, and its position within the uterus. The myometrium and cervix should be evaluated for contour changes, echogenicity, and masses.

C. ADNEXA (OVARIES AND FALLOPIAN TUBES)

- When evaluating the adnexa, an attempt should be made to identify the ovaries first since they can serve as the major point of reference for adnexal structures.

Frequently the ovaries are situated anterior to the internal iliac (hypogastric) vessels, which serve as landmarks for their identification. The following ovarian findings should be documented: size and position relative to the uterus. The ovarian size can be determined by measuring the length in long axis with the anteroposterior dimension measured perpendicular to the length. The ovarian width is measured in the transaxial or coronal view. A volume can be calculated.

• The normal fallopian tubes are not commonly identified. This region should be surveyed for abnormalities, particularly dilated tubular structures. If an adnexal mass is noted, its relationship to the ovaries and uterus should be documented. Its size and echo pattern (cystic, solid, or mixed) should be determined. A search for embryonic cardiac activity should be conducted when appropriate. Doppler or color Doppler ultrasound may be useful in select cases and can identify the vascular nature of tubular pelvic structures.

D. CUL-DE-SAC

• The cul-de-sac and bowel posterior to the uterus may not be clearly defined. This area should be evaluated for the presence of free fluid or a mass. If a mass is detected, its size, position, shape, echo pattern (cystic, solid, or complex), and relationship to the ovaries and uterus should be documented. Differentiation of normal loops of bowel from a mass may be difficult if only an abdominal examination is performed. A transvaginal examination may be helpful to distinguish a suspected mass from fluid and feces within the normal rectosigmoid. An ultrasound water enema study or a repeat examination after a cleansing enema may also help distinguish a suspected mass from bowel.

IV. DOCUMENTATION

• Adequate documentation is essential for high-quality patient care. There should be a permanent record of the ultrasound examination and its interpretation included in the medical record. Images of all appropriate areas, both normal and abnormal, should be recorded in an image or storage format. Variations from normal size should be accompanied by measurements. Images are to be appropriately labeled with the examination date, facility name, patient identification, date of last menstrual period or relevant menopausal history, image orientation, and, whenever possible, the organ or area imaged. Retention of the permanent record of the ultrasound examination should be consistent with both clinical need and the relevant legal and local healthcare facility requirements. Reporting should be in accordance with the ACR Standard for Communication: Diagnostic Radiology.

V. EQUIPMENT

• Ultrasound examination of the female pelvis should be conducted with a real-time scanner, preferably using sector, curved linear, or endovaginal transducers. The transducer or scanner should be adjusted to operate at the highest clinically appropriate frequency, realizing that there is a trade-off between resolution and beam penetration.

• With modern equipment, studies performed from the anterior abdominal wall can usually use frequencies of 3.5 MHz or higher, while scans performed from the vagina should use frequencies of 5 MHz or higher. All probes should be cleaned after use. Vaginal probes should be covered by a protective sheath prior to insertion. Following the examination, the sheath should be disposed of and the probe cleaned in an antimicrobial solution. The type of solution and amount of time for cleaning depends on manufacturer and infectious disease recommendations.

VI. QUALITY CONTROL AND IMPROVEMENT, SAFETY, INFECTION CONTROL, AND PATIENT EDUCATION CONCERNS

• Policies and procedures related to quality, patient education, infection control, and safety should be developed and implemented in accordance with the ACR Policy on Quality Control and Improvement, Safety, Infection Control, and Patient Education Concerns appearing elsewhere in the ACR Standards Book.

• Equipment performance monitoring should be in accordance with the ACR Standard for Diagnostic Medical Physics Performance Monitoring of Real-Time B-Mode Ultrasound Equipment.

Appendix 2
American College of Radiology (ACR) Standard for the Performance of Antepartum Obstetrical Ultrasound

I. INTRODUCTION

- These guidelines have been developed for use by practitioners performing obstetrical ultrasound studies. Fetal ultrasound should be performed only when there is a valid medical reason, and the lowest possible ultrasonic exposure settings should be used to gain the necessary diagnostic information. A limited examination may be performed in clinical emergencies or used as a follow-up to a complete examination. In some cases, additional and/or specialized examinations may be necessary. While it is not possible to detect all structural congenital anomalies with diagnostic ultrasound, adherence to the following guidelines will maximize the possibility of detecting many fetal abnormalities.

II. QUALIFICATIONS AND RESPONSIBILITIES OF THE PHYSICIAN

- See the ACR Standard for Performing and Interpreting Diagnostic Ultrasound Examinations.

III. SPECIFICATIONS OF THE EXAMINATION

A. FIRST-TRIMESTER SONOGRAPHY

1. INDICATIONS
- An ultrasound examination can be of benefit in many circumstances in the first trimester of pregnancy, including, but not limited to, the following indications:
a. To confirm the presence of an intrauterine pregnancy.
b. To evaluate a suspected ectopic pregnancy.
c. To define the cause of vaginal bleeding of undetermined etiology.
d. To estimate gestational age.
e. To confirm suspected multiple gestations.
f. To confirm embryonic life.
g. As an adjunct to chorionic villus sampling, amniocentesis, embryo transfer, and intrauterine device (IUD) localization and removal.
h. To evaluate pelvic masses.
i. To detect uterine abnormalities.
   Comment
   - Limited examination may be performed to follow up growth, estimate amniotic fluid, check cervical length, and assess viability.

2. GUIDELINES
- *Overall Comment:* Scanning in the first trimester may be performed either abdominally or vaginally. If a transabdominal examination is performed and fails to provide definitive information concerning any of the following guidelines, a transvaginal scan should be done whenever possible.
a. The uterus and adnexa should be evaluated for the presence of a gestational sac. If a gestational sac is seen, its location should be documented. The presence or absence of an embryo should be noted and the crown-rump length recorded.
   Comments
   - The crown-rump length is a more accurate indicator of gestational age than is gestational sac diameter. Comparison should be made to standard tables.
   - If the embryo is not identified, the mean diameter of the gestational sac should be calculated to estimate gestational age and the gestational sac should be evaluated for presence and size of the yolk sac.
   - Caution should be used in making the presumptive diagnosis of a gestational sac in the absence of a definite fetal pole or yolk sac, because without these findings an intrauterine fluid collection could represent a pseudogestational sac associated with an ectopic pregnancy.

255

- While not considered part of the minimum required examination, it is desirable to examine other areas of fetal anatomy when fetal position permits. Such views can at times be difficult to obtain because of fetal lie, amniotic fluid level, and maternal body habitus.
- Suspected abnormalities may require an in-depth evaluation of the area(s) of concern.

IV. DOCUMENTATION

- Adequate documentation of the study is essential for high-quality patient care. This should include a permanent record of the ultrasound images, incorporating whenever possible the measurement parameters and anatomical findings proposed in this document. Images should be appropriately labeled with the examination date, patient identification, and, if appropriate, image orientation. A written report of the ultrasound findings should be included in the patient's medical record. Reporting should be in accordance with the ACR Standard for Communication: Diagnostic Radiology. Retention of the ultrasound examination should be consistent with both clinical need and relevant legal and local healthcare facility requirements.

V. EQUIPMENT SPECIFICATIONS

- These studies should be conducted with real-time scanners, using a transabdominal and/or transvaginal approach. A transducer of appropriate frequency should be used.

Comments
- Real time is necessary to confirm the presence of fetal life through observation of cardiac activity and active movement.
- The choice of transducer frequency is a trade-off between beam penetration and resolution. With modern equipment, 3- to 5-MHz abdominal transducers allow sufficient penetration in most patients while providing adequate resolution. A lower-frequency transducer (2 to 2.25 MHz) may be needed to provide adequate penetration for abdominal imaging in an obese patient. During early pregnancy, a 5-MHz abdominal or a 5- to 7.5-MHz vaginal transducer may provide superior resolution while still allowing adequate penetration.

VI. QUALITY CONTROL AND IMPROVEMENT, SAFETY, INFECTION CONTROL, AND PATIENT EDUCATION CONCERNS

- Policies and procedures related to quality, patient education, infection control, and safety should be developed and implemented in accordance with the ACR Policy on Quality Control and Improvement, Safety, Infection Control, and Patient Education Concerns appearing elsewhere in the ACR Standards Book.
- Equipment performance monitoring should be in accordance with the ACR Standard for Diagnostic Medical Physics Performance Monitoring of Real Time B-Mode Ultrasound Equipment.

INDEX

INDEX

A

Abdominal disorders, in fetus, 203
Abdominal ectopic pregnancy, 162. *See also* Ectopic pregnancy
Abortion
  completed, 178f
  missed. *See* Pregnancy, failed
Abruption placenta, 205
Accreditation, 3
Achondroplastic dwarf, 204
Adenomyosis
  CDS of, 125f
  definition of, 36
  TV-CDS findings of, 117
  TVS of, 35
Adhesions, SHG of, 132, 146f
Adnexal torsion
  CDS of, 121f, 122f
  degrees of, 119f
  detection of, 96
  during pregnancy, 237
  TV-CDS of, 117, 120f, 122f
  TVS of, 117
American College of Radiology (ACR)
  accreditation by, 3
  standards for antepartum ultrasound, 255–258
  standards for ultrasound examination of pelvis, 253–254
American Institute of Ultrasound in Medicine (AIUM),
    accreditation by, 3
Amniocentesis
  in early pregnancy, 163
  in mid- to late pregnancy, 201, 202
Amniotic fluid assessment, 202, 214f
Amniotic fluid index (AFI), 202
Anteflexed uterus, 35
  TVS of, 37f
Aortic arch, 220f
  CDS of, 221f
Appendiceal abscess, TVS of, 115f
Appendicitis, 237
  as cause of pelvic pain, 118
  CDS of, 238f
  TA-CDS of, 128f
  TV-CDS of, 118
Archiving
  film *vs.* paper images, 3
  types of, 3

Arrhythmias, in fetus, 203
Artifacts
  multiple reverberation, 7f
  side lobe, 7f
  types of, 2
Asherman's syndrome, 74f
Asymmetric IUGR, 202
Axial resolution, 1, 6f

B

Balloon catheter, in SHG, 74f
Bicornuate uterus, 35
  TAS of, 45f
Bioeffects, definition of, 1
Biophysical profile scoring, for fetus, 206t
Biparietal diameter, measurement of, 201, 209f
Breast carcinoma, 243f
  SonoCT image of, 245f
Breast cyst, 242f
  during needle aspiration, 244f
Breast masses, during pregnancy, 237
Breast sonogram, performance of, 244f

C

Cardiac anomalies, in fetus, 203
Catheters
  balloon, 74f
  Foley, 74f
  H/S, 71f
  Soules insemination, 75f
  Tampa, 71f
Central nervous system anomalies
  assessment of, 215f
  in fetus, 202–203
Cervical ectopic pregnancy, 162. *See also*
    Ectopic pregnancy
Cervical fibroids. *See* Fibroids
Cervix, 18f–21f
  incompetence of, 207
  length of, 236f
  normal configuration of, 207
  transvaginal sonogram of, 236f
Chorionic sac, TVS of, 168f
Chorionic villus sampling (CVS), 163, 199f

K

Kidneys
  hydronephrotic, 225f
  normal view, 223f

L

Late pregnancy. *See* Pregnancy, late
Lateral resolution, 1, 6f
Leiomyomas. *See* Fibroids
Leiomyosarcoma, 36
  photomicrograph of, 48f
Limb anomalies, in fetus, 204
Linear array transvaginal probes, 1, 5f
Linear phased array, 6f
Linear sequenced array, 6f
Lungs, cystic adenomatoid malformations in, 203, 219f

M

Magnetic resonance imaging (MRI), in evaluation of uterine
    shape, 131
Maternal bowel disorders, 129f
Mechanical index (MI), 3
Mechanical sector probes, 1
Meckel-Gruber syndrome, 204
Meconium peritonitis, 203, 223f
Meningomyelocele, 202, 204
Menometrorrhagia
  progestin as treatment for, 83f
  SHG of, 83f
Mid-pregnancy. *See* Pregnancy, middle
Molar pregnancy, 163
Monochorionic gestation, 162
Monochorionic twins, 228f
Mucinous cystadenoma, 102f, 103f
Multicystic displastic kidney, 224f, 227f
  in fetus, 204
Multifetal pregnancy, 162
  TVS of, 175f
Multiparous uterus, 15, 35
Myometrium, vascular invasion of, 230f
Myxomatous uterine tumor, TAS of, 110f

N

Native Tissue Harmonic Imaging, 8f, 9f
Near field/far field resolution, 2
Neck anomalies, in fetus, 203
Needle aspiration, TVS guidance for, 144f
Nuchal translucency, 163
  TVS of, 197f, 198f
Nulliparous uterus, 15

O

Omphalocele, 222f
  vs. gastroschisis, 203
Ostia, identification of, 79f

Ovarian cancer
  and breast cancer, 132
  CDS detection of, 132
  risk factors for, 132
  screening for, 132
  3D Doppler scan of, 251f
  TV-CDS of, 116f
  TVS of, 105f, 106f, 132
Ovarian ectopic pregnancy, 162. *See also*
    Ectopic Pregnancy
Ovarian hyperstimulation syndrome, 131
  TVS of, 138f–139f
Ovarian masses, 95
  CDS of, 96
  diagnosis of, 96
  identification of, 96
  sonographic appearance of, 97
Ovarian tumors
  with abnormal arterial waveforms, 150f
  arrangement of vessels, 116f
  early stage, 149f
  growth *vs.* vascularity, 156f
  stage II, 149f
  TV-CDS of, 148f–150f
  vascularity network of, 157f
Ovarian vein thrombosis, as cause of pelvic pain, 118
Ovaries
  ACR standards for sonography of, 253–254
  CDS of, 31f
  size and shape of, 16
  torsion of, 117, 119f–121f, 121f
  TVS of, 22f, 30f, 32f
  vasculature of, 31f, 157f

P

Papillary excrescences, as evidence of
    malignancy, 96
Parous uterus
  adult, 40f
  postmenopausal, 40f
Pedunculated fibroids, 36, 46f
Pelvic congestion, 117
  TV-CDS of, 127f
Pelvic examination
  ACR standards for, 253–254
  documentation of, 254
  equipment for, 254
  and quality control, 254
Pelvic hematoma, TVS of, 112f
Pelvic masses
  assessment for regression in, 95
  benign, 96t
  caused by tubal disorders, 96
  complex, 95t, 98f
  cystic, 95t
    right adrenal, 99f
    TAS of, 99f
    transverse TAS of, 102f

TV-CDS of, 154f–155f
TVS of, 99f–101f, 104f, 153f
differential diagnosis of, 95t
features of, 95
location of, 95, 98f
malignant, 96t
during pregnancy, 237
solid, 95t
    interligamentous fibroid as, 109f
    transverse TAS of, 109t
    TVS of, 107f
TAS of, 95
TV-CDS of, 238f
TVS of, 103f
Pelvic organs, 98f
Pelvic pain
    and adnexal torsion, 117
    from appendicitis, 118
    from irritable bowel syndrome, 118
    from ovarian causes, 118
    sonographic evaluation of, 117, 237
    from ureteral calculi, 118
    uterine causes of, 117
Phased array transvaginal probes, 5f
Philips/ATL 4000 scanner, 11f
Picture archive communication system (PACS), 3
Placenta
    abnormal implantation, 205
    abnormal location, 204–205
    blood flow from, 228f
    cross section of, 165f
    disorders of, 204–205
    normal function of, 205
Placenta previa, 204
Polyps, 58
    SHG of, 131
Postmenopausal bleeding, 57
    TVS of, 58, 68f
Postmenopausal uterus, 15, 35
    TAS of, 40f
    TVS of, 40f
Postmenstrual endometrium, SHG of, 82f
Post-pubertal uterus, 15, 35
    TAS of, 39f
    TVS of, 39f
Potter's syndrome, 204
Power, in spectral analysis, 2
Pregnancy
    early
        ACR guidelines for sonography during,
            255–256
        complications of, 176f
        diagnostic procedures in, 163
        TAS of, 167f
        TVS of, 167f–169f
        uterine vessels in, 171f
    ectopic. *See* Ectopic pregnancy
    failed, 162
        TVS of, 176f

late
    ACR guidelines for sonography during, 256–258
    common problems in, 201
    definition of, 201
middle
    ACR guidelines for sonography during, 256–258
    common problems in, 201
    definition of, 201
molar, 163
Pre-pubertal uterus, 15, 35
Probes
    definition of, 1
    transabdominal, 1
    transvaginal, 1, 5f
Pseudocyst, TVS of, 113f
Pseudomembranous colitis, sonogram of, 129f
Pulsatility index (P.I.), 2

R
Renal agenesis, bilateral, 204, 224f
Renal anomalies, in fetus, 203
Renal calculi, 237
Resistive index (R.I.), 2
Resolution
    factors affecting, 1–2
    techniques for improvement in, 2
    types of, 1–2
Retrochorionic hemorrhage, 161, 162
    TVS of, 177f
Retroflexed uterus, 35
    endometrium in, 61f
    TVS of, 37f
Reverberation artifacts, 2

S
Scanner memory, 2
Scanning technique, 3
Sector array probes, 1
Septated uterus, 35
Side lobe artifacts, 2
Small bowel, 33f
SonoCT technique, 2, 10f
Sonography
    bioeffects considerations in, 3
    contrast-enhanced, 247
    definition of, 1
    role in fetal development, 201–207
    technique, 3
    versatility of, 247
Sonohysterography (SHG)
    of adhesions, 132
    catheters for, 38f, 74f
    for evaluation of tubal patency, 59
    findings, 59
    with H/S catheter, 73f
    in infertility, 145f
    instrumentation, 71f

Sonohysterography (SHG) (*cont.*)
   long- and short-axis images, 78f
   of patent tubes, 142f–143f
   of polyps, 131
   procedure, 58
   scanning maneuvers in, 72f
   scan planes used for, 77f
   of submucosal fibroids, 131
   technique, 58–59, 71f
   use of positive microbubble contrast with, 59
Sonosalpingography, diagram of, 140f
Soules insemination catheter, 75f
Spectral analysis, 2
Spina bifida, 226f
Spinal anomalies, in fetus, 204, 226f
Spiral arteries, transformation during pregnancy, 236f
Submucosal fibroids, 36, 46f
   SHG of, 131
   SHG of in, 147f
Subserosal fibroids, 36, 46f
Succenturiate lobe, 205, 229f
Symmetric IUGR, 202
Synechiae, sonohysterogram of, 91

T
Tamoxifen therapy, 51f
   for breast cancer, 58
   TVS of, 70f
Tampa catheter, 71f
Thanatophoric dysplasia, 226f
Thanatotophoric dwarf, 204
Thermal index (TI), 3
Three-dimensional color Doppler sonography (3D-CDS)
   for assessing fibroid vascularity, 36
   of fibroids, 49f
Three-dimensional sonography
   appropriateness of, 247
   availability of, 247
   of fetal anatomy, 248f
   of uterine malformation, 46f
   of uterus, 249f
Tight convex probes, 1
Time gain compensation (TGC), 2
Toshiba, Aplio scanner, 11f
Transabdominal sonography (TAS)
   of enlarged uterus, 9f
   for pelvic masses, 95
   for providing global overview, 15
   scanning planes used with, 17f
   technique of, 3
Transducers
   definition of, 1
   design of, 2
Transperineal scans, 3
Transrectal sonography (TRS), 3
   and circlage placement, 55f
   diagram of, 53f
   in dilatation and curettage, 36, 54f

Transvaginal color Doppler sonography (TV-CDS), 42f
   of endometrial disorders, 92f
   frequency-based, 116f
   in tumor detection, 148f–150f
   of uterine bleeding, 94f
Transvaginal sonography (TVS)
   ALARA principle used with, 161
   in diagnosis of adenomyosis, 36
   in early pregnancy, 161
   in evaluation of fibroids, 36
   in evaluation of uterine shape, 131
   in fertility disorders, 131
   for intrauterine pregnancy, 161
   and postmenopausal bleeding, 58
   for providing detailed depiction, 15
   technique, 3, 14f, 15, 35
Tubal patency, 131
   contrast enhancement for, 247
   TVS of, 141f
Tubal torsion, CDS of, 124f
Tumor angiogenesis, 157f
Tumor vascularity, contrast enhancement for, 247

U
Ultrasound. *See* Sonography
Ultrasound PACS display module, 14f
Umbilical artery, flow velocity waveforms,
     229f, 231f
Umbilical cord
   anomalies of, 205
   CDS of, 234f
   development of, 232f
   normal function of, 205
   sonographic image of, 233f
Unilateral renal agenesis, 224f
Ureteral calculi, as cause of pelvic pain, 118
Ureteral stones, locations of, 118
Ureteropelvic junction (UPJ) obstruction,
     204, 225f
Uterine artery, CDS of, 235f
Uterine bleeding
   dysfunctional, 58, 66f
   and endometrium disorders, 57
Uterine cervix. *See* Cervix
Uterine cornua, 33f
Uterine malformation, 3D sonography of, 46f, 143f
Uterine malformations, sonography of, 35
Uterine masses. *See* Fibroids
Uterine shape, evaluation of, 131
Uterine vascularity, transvaginal color Doppler sonography
     (TV-CDS) of, 43f
Uterus
   ACR standards for sonography of, 253
   anteflexed, 20f, 23f, 35, 37f
   bicornuate, 35, 45f
   blood supply to, 23f, 24f, 136f, 235f
   configuration of, 15, 35, 39f
   flexion of, 35

long axis view of, 18f, 22f, 39f
malformations of, 35, 45f
myometrial layers of, 15, 24f
normal sonographic anatomy, 35, 41f
nulliparous, 15
parous, 40f
pre-pubertal, 15, 35
retroflexed, 20f, 21f, 23f, 35
   endometrium in, 61f
    TVS of, 37f
short axis view of, 22f, 39f
3D sonography of, 249f
transabdominal sonogram of, 37f
TVS of, 18f–21f, 38f

V
Vasa previa, 205
Video, for image storage, 3

X
XRes algorithm, 2
XRes technology, 10f

Y
Yolk sac, 161
   progressive growth of, 166f
   transvaginal sonogram of, 169f